Foods for Moods

To Fiorella

Foods for Moods

William Vayda

**GEDDES &
GROSSET**

This edition published 2007 by Geddes & Grosset,
David Dale House, New Lanark, ML11 9DJ, Scotland
First published in this edition 2004, reprinted 2007

First published in Australia in 1992 by Thomas C. Lothian Pty Ltd

ISBN 978 1 84205 351 5

Printed and bound in Poland

POLSKABOOK

CONTENTS

ACKNOWLEDGEMENTS

My gratitude goes to three of the most brilliant minds in psychiatry. The true pioneers, Dr Richard Mackarness, Dr Abraham Hoffer and Dr Bernard Rimland, who have inspired and informed me. From them I learned the twin principles of nutritional psychiatry and clinical ecology. I would also like to thank the many Australian scientists and doctors who have contributed to and helped with my knowledge and experience.

ABOUT THE AUTHOR

William Vayda, one of Australia's pioneers in orthomolecular medicine and psychiatry, specialises in nutritional and environmental medicine. He is particularly involved in the treatment of chronic fatigue, post-viral syndromes and disorders of immunity, especially allergic syndromes (asthma, candida, arthritis), and psychiatric disorders related to nutritional problems.

A graduate osteopath, William Vayda first became interested in the role of nutrition in psychiatry and obtained post-graduate diplomas in nutrition-naturopathy, acupuncture and clinical hypnotherapy.

He was appointed senior lecturer in physiology and nutrition at the Sydney College of Chiropractic and Osteopathy in 1973 and later taught differential diagnosis and clinical nutrition. The following year he founded the Australian Institute for Orthomolecular Research in Sydney.

In the late 1970s, he ran a training programme for medical doctors and other health professionals and ran special post-graduate courses in nutritional and environmental medicine and psychiatry, thus providing the impetus towards a complementary approach to medicine in Australia.

Working as a clinician and diagnostician with a group of open-minded and progressive medical scientists, he carried out extensive research into the role of nutrition in mental illness and the role of allergies and chemicals in asthma and immunological disorders.

William Vayda is president of the International College of

Applied Nutrition (Australia), and a fellow of the Oceania College of Clinical Nutrition. He is a member of the International Association of Orthomolecular Medicine, the Australasian Society of Osteopaths, the Complementary Medicine Association, the International Academy of Preventative Medicine, the Academy of Orthomolecular Psychiatry, the Huxley Institute for Bio-Social Research, the New York Academy of Science and the Australian Natural Therapists Association (ANTA).

He has lectured extensively at universities, medical schools, various naturopathic colleges and to the general public. He is a well-known and prolific writer of popular columns and scientific papers. He had a weekly health column in the Sydney *Sun* newspaper for many years and was nutrition/science editor of *Nature and Health* magazine for several years. He is now a contributing editor of *Wellbeing* magazine and has written several best-selling books. These include the following:

Health for Life: Are you Allergic to the 20th Century ?
The Candida Questions and Answers Book
Chronic Fatigue, the Silent Epidemic

INTRODUCTION

Psycho-nutrition is the popular name given to the branch of medicine that deals with nutrition and its effect on the mind. This branch of medicine, orthomolecular psychiatry, looks at the effects of natural chemicals, such as vitamins, minerals and amino acids, on the brain's chemistry.

In the 1950s, two psychiatrists, Dr Abraham Hoffer and his colleague Dr Osmond, discovered that certain people showed signs of mental illness if they were deficient in Vitamin B$_3$ (niacin), and that other people's mental illnesses could be helped by administering large amounts of certain nutrients that were either deficient in their diet or for which these individuals had unusually high requirements. Both groups using nutritional therapy improved considerably and many individuals completely recovered.

Even though the niacin treatment was successful and a great deal less harmful than the standard psychiatric regimen of the 1950s (electro convulsive therapy (ECT), insulin shock and psychoactive drugs) the orthodox scientific community was, and still is, slow to acknowledge these findings. Many great scientists, including Nobel prize winner Linus Pauling (who in 1968 wrote a memorable article titled 'Orthomolecular Psychiatry' for *Science*), were looking for more links between nutrition and mental illness. Within a few years a host of vitamins and several minerals were found to help the niacin treatment and so orthomolecular psychiatry became a complex therapy involving a formidable array of nutrients.

At the same time, other workers in the field discovered that fluctuations in blood sugar (hypoglycaemia), which could occur independently of vitamin deficiencies, were also capable of causing a number of physical and mental disorders which mimicked many psychiatric conditions. Many patients regained their health as a result of understanding that diet, as well as vitamins and minerals, could influence mental health.

Dr Richard Mackarness, a psychiatrist at Basingstoke District Hospital in England, had studied and applied the findings of Dr Theodore Randolph, a leader in the study of allergies, to mentally ill patients. After much success with nutritional therapy, Dr Mackarness wrote a book called *Not all in the Mind* which was first published in England in 1976. For the first time the average person, as well as professionals in the field of psychiatry, could read a simple yet shattering account of diagnostic and treatment methods which were brilliant in both their simplicity and effectiveness.

Psychiatry and our understanding of human behaviour and brain biochemistry took a giant leap forward: we learned that while vitamin and mineral deficiencies, or dependencies, still played a major role in orthomolecular psychiatry, it was pointless running blood tests for vitamin deficiencies or glucose tolerance tests for hypoglycaemics when we could first find out if they were hypersensitive (allergic or intolerant) to some foods, certain chemicals or even airborne environmental factors. Any of these hypersensitivities could be 'causing' nutritional imbalances and deficiencies by promoting malabsorption; they could equally 'cause' hypoglycaemia by placing such a stress on the body's ability to cope that blood sugar levels would plummet anyway!

Later, we discovered that an overgrowth of candida albicans (candidiasis) could also cause, or be caused by, any or all of the above factors and so it became more and more obvious that we had to start by eliminating what was the major factor at hand at present rather than the underlying cause. For example, if hypoglycaemia were causing someone to be stressed and this manifested as an allergy which allowed candida organisms to grow unchecked, we have to start treating the overgrowing bugs (or the presenting symptoms). Once they are taken care of, then the allergies and blood-sugar problems should be dealt with. If the problems do not improve then we should look for any independent 'causes'.

Perhaps as a legacy from orthodox medicine, some people still have difficulty accepting that it is quite possible for a psychiatric patient to suffer brain-chemistry dysfunction caused by a deficiency of niacin while also being hypoglycaemic because of diet—without the two being necessarily related in a cause-and-effect continuum. While correcting the hypoglycaemia with diet will make him or her healthier, the psychiatric problem will not be taken care of until supplementary niacin is given. Conversely, treating the vitamin problem and the hypoglycaemia as well as the food allergies or intolerances may not ensure good health while the patient is exposed to airborne moulds or dust.

One promising nutritional treatment, known as 'precursor therapy', is now routinely employed by all of us in treating candidiasis and yeast-related problems. Precursor therapy makes use of pure amino acids which are the precursors of most, if not all, of the brain chemicals or neurotransmitters which control our moods. For example, a patient with allergies or an infection, such as candidiasis, may also suffer with depression. In such a case, the administration of an amino acid, such as DL-phenylalanine, or perhaps L-tyrosine, will reduce depression while the treatment for the other condition is carried out. This is possible because both amino acids are precursors of brain chemicals that act naturally as anti-depressants.

It is the ability to keep an open mind that has characterised many of the great scientists and it is my hope that this book not only informs a great many readers but also encourages all of us, including the orthodox medical community, to keep an open mind and to look for better, more simple and less harmful ways to help our fellow humans.

1

MEMORY—HOW TO IMPROVE IT AND THINK CLEARLY

If you wish to maximise your brain functions, including memory, it would be a good idea to start by learning something about how the brain works.

How the brain works

The human brain is an irregular globe of moist, jelly-like tissue containing more than ten billion nerve cells called 'neurons'. Each neuron has numerous root-like fibres with tiny bulbs at the ends. Minute amounts of chemicals burst out of these bulbs continually, and hit the walls of other brain cells. Once these other cells are charged they fire their own chemicals, and this activity is repeated millions of times each minute of our lives. These chemicals are known as neurotransmitters.

Learning, memory, moods, sleep, appetite and sex drive are all controlled by neurotransmitters. In fact, we literally cannot make a move without them because they also control the co-ordination of our muscles.

We also have controllers of these controls: more chemicals. We are not sure what they all are but we do know that diet does influence the type and amount of neurotransmitters. Vitamins and minerals are involved, in fact essential, in the production of these brain chemicals from ordinary amino acids extracted from the proteins in our daily food.

There are some thirty known neurotransmitters and probably many more that we don't yet know about and all of them are made from amino acids. Food is broken down into individual amino acids which then enter brain cells and are converted to neurotransmitters in a series of biochemical steps which cannot take place without the presence of several essential vitamins and minerals. That is why it is possible to treat emotional and psychiatric problems with highly individualised diets and nutrients such as vitamins and amino acids.

If someone is allergic, hypersensitive or has an intolerance to some foods or the chemicals which they contain, these can cause the brain to react adversely and therefore cause a sort of 'brain-allergy' reaction.

Placing such patients on a diet that avoids these sensitising foods or chemicals can often cure, or greatly help, their condition. However, in many cases, simply changing a diet so that it includes the appropriate amino acids for the required neurotransmitters does not work satisfactorily. That is why we usually prescribe amino acids as supplements (precursor therapy).

Dietary manipulations do not work satisfactorily because most foods contain a number of amino acids and they all compete to get to the brain. As there are only a limited number of 'seats' on the blood-to-brain bus (see 'The blood-brain barrier' below), too many amino acids of one kind will stop others from even getting on the bus.

For example, turkey contains lots of tryptophan (an amino acid the brain turns into serotonin) which makes you sleep well. Many similar foods contain an excess of 'competing' amino acids and eating them will give little benefit if eaten at bedtime in order to treat insomnia.

If, however, you take some carbohydrates at the same time (say a tablespoon of honey) this will help to elevate blood sugar and that inevitably causes the release of insulin which has the unusual effect of chasing away several amino acids from the blood into the liver. Insulin does not, however, affect tryptophan so that now this amino acid has the bus to the brain all to itself and there is a good chance you will then get a good night's sleep.

PRECURSORS

Precursors are the substances, in this case a dietary or supplemental amino acid, from which the brain makes a neurotransmitter. Following is a short list of some of the amino acids and the main neurotransmitters that are derived from them.

Source/Precursor	Neurotransmitter
choline/serine	acetylcholine
histidine	histamine
tyrosine	epinephrine, norepinephrine
phenylalanine	tyrosine, dopamine, norepinephrine
tryptophan	serotonin
glutamic acid	glutamine/gamma aminobutyric acid (GABA)
lysine	citrulline, pipecolic acid

As you can see, it is not enough to know what to eat. You must also know when to eat and how to combine your food if you want to influence brain chemistry via diet. This, of course, is something we all do on a daily basis without ever realising it.

The answer is not simply taking amino acids (as supplements) because they will not always work and, in some cases, they can make matters worse. The key is to take only those supplements that are needed for particular individuals depending on their specific circumstances. This applies to almost every diet, pill or potion but especially so to anything that may act on your brain.

We are all biochemically unique and what may put one person to sleep, may keep another awake all night. This, for instance, can happen with tryptophan if you happen to be a heavy drinker.

The blood-brain barrier

As cells go, neurons are particularly frail. Their functions can be disrupted by an incredibly large number of toxic substances and 'natural' molecules, such as amino acids, that are normally present in the blood but kept away from the brain's own private circulation.

Folic acid, for example, a nutrient regarded as a vitamin, is essential for the body's good health. Normally, however, very little folic acid is allowed to pass from the blood stream into the brain's circulation. When too much folic acid does enter the brain, it can cause convulsions and, in fact, a group of drugs used for the treatment of epilepsy act precisely as antifolates.

A complex barrier has evolved in the human brain to keep it isolated from general circulation. This selective filtration system, known as the blood-brain barrier, normally allows only oxygen, glucose and a few selected nutrients to penetrate it. While the knowledge of how the blood-brain barrier works is invaluable in designing drugs that will act on specific neuron complexes, it is equally important in deciding which nutrient may play a role in altering brain functions.

Psychobiologists have discovered that the behavioural effects of many drugs, neurotoxins and 'foreign' molecules occur precisely because of their ability to disrupt, or modify, the orderly chemical transmission between neurons. We also know that 'mental illnesses' may be caused by excessive, insufficient, imbalanced or defective neurotransmitters. And practically all these neurotransmitters are made from common constituents of the foods we eat every day.

Nutrients for the brain

Despite its relatively small size, the human brain consumes more energy than any other organ. Representing only 2 per cent of total body weight, the brain uses 20 per cent of the total resting oxygen of the body.

Everyone knows that the brain cannot function without oxygen and that brain damage follows after even a small period of time without it. However, what must be understood is the underlying reason why oxygen is crucial to brain function. Oxygen is needed to make glucose available which is the primary source of all brain energy. If the flow of oxygenated blood to the brain is interrupted an individual will lose consciousness within 10 seconds. A little longer may cause permanent brain damage. It is also worthwhile to note

CUDDLES AND BRAIN POWER

Intelligence, brain power, memory and just about every activity the brain performs are greatly dependent on the formation of new connections. In addition, the protein content of each cell is constantly being destroyed and remade.

This building activity is largely dependent on the stimulation of nerve fibres (input equals action potential) which occurs whenever our central nervous system is busy.

Even just touching, stroking or cuddling a child can have an enormous impact on its future intelligence potential. Babies deprived of physical contact have fewer neuron connections and may become mentally and physically stunted.

There is, in fact, a well documented syndrome called 'deprivation dwarfism' caused by a lack of sensory inputs to an infant. 'If you don't use it you'll lose it' is an old adage which applies equally to brain power as it does to libido, memory and muscular strength.

that similar effects can be caused by any condition that lowers blood-sugar levels (these are discussed under 'Hypoglycaemia' on page 48).

A prerequisite for optimal brain power is, therefore, a good supply of oxygen which is transported to the brain by the blood. Good blood flow is critical if we are to use our brain efficiently.

There are many ways to improve your circulation: regular exercise and special yoga positions can influence it; a good massage given by expert hands can enhance your circulation; chiropractic manipulations can free previously restricted blood supply to the brain by correcting spinal and neck sub-luxations; and all reputable acupuncturists know several points that help the body maintain a healthy blood flow. In addition to physical methods of increasing circulation, there are several nutrients that also play a role, such as Vitamin E, Vitamin B_3 (niacin) and ginseng.

Because blood sugar supplies are so critical to brain functions, you should ensure that glucose levels in the brain are not allowed to fall too far, or too rapidly. A condition known as hypoglycaemia (low blood sugar) can play havoc with anyone trying to think clearly. Two of the most common causes of hypoglycaemia are unsuspected food allergies or intolerances and candidiasis (systemic thrush). Another syndrome which often appears simultaneously with low blood-sugar levels, and may either be its cause or one of its effects, is hypoadrenocorticism, or exhausted adrenal glands.

Nutrition plays a central role in the treatment of all these conditions and so chemicals which the brain uses to make its own special foods, and which are readily available in your diet, are a good place to start looking for ways to improve your brain. Adhere to a well-balanced diet with a reasonable amount of proteins, some complex carbohydrates, no refined sugars or sweets and small, frequent snacks rather than few large meals.

The two memory banks

It has been proposed that memory is stored in two different parts of the brain: one that records events for a relatively short period of time (known as short-term memory bank) and a long-term memory into which events from the first bank are transferred. Unless information is transferred from the short to the long-term memory bank within a specified period, it is lost forever.

In the late 1940s, Donald Hebb, a psychologist at McGill University in Montreal, proposed that when neurons receive repeated stimulation from nerve cells they become more and more sensitive to the signals with the result that information becomes encoded in the more permanent memory. We all know that by repeating information, say a telephone number, we are more likely to remember it. Today we still don't know how the brain remembers, let alone where the memories are stored, but Hebb's theories remain the best explanation we have.

There are several factors which can interfere with memory. Several commonly used drugs are known to affect memory adversely. Lorazepam, a tranquilliser, can be used to help people forget unhappy experiences. Ovobain, a digitalis-like drug used in the treatment of heart disease, interferes with the electrical impulses in the brain that are necessary for memory storage and may also inhibit the synthesis of proteins with which memory is thought to be encoded. Whatever the reason, another drug, an antibiotic called Puromycin,

THE HIPPOCAMPUS

By 1973, Tim Bliss, of the National Institute for Medical Research in London, and Terje Lomo, of the Institute of Neurophysiology at the University of Oslo in Norway, narrowed their research on memory to a part of the brain known as the hippocampus. This small structure is believed to be essential for memory.

Certainly we know that even lower vertebrates can learn provided they have a hippocampus and that invertebrates, which have no hippocampus, are unable to learn. Scientists have demonstrated that repeated electrical stimulation over long periods of time of hippocampal neurons makes brain cells more sensitive to stimulation.

The brains of people suffering from alcohol-induced damage can often be seen to have impaired hippocampal functions and, according to several orthomolecular scientists, zinc deficiencies can render this portion of the brain inefficient.

Whether taking zinc supplements can increase memory remains to be seen. However, we do already know that zinc (which reduces brain levels of copper which excite brain cells) can produce a degree of mental relaxation, reduce lead accumulation and improve the conditions of some schizophrenics and alcoholics.

has been shown to wipe out long-term memory, and its mode of action is that of blocking protein synthesis.

It would seem that any drug which affects the central nervous system, whether a tranquilliser, narcotic, sedative, analgesic or antipsychotic, has the potential to influence human memory adversely.

Serotonin and tryptophan

Serotonin is associated with sleep, moods and perception. Too little serotonin may cause sleeplessness, depression and difficulties with temperature regulation. Too much may be involved with premature ageing, psychosis, sleeplessness and aggressive behaviour. Although no direct connection between serotonin and memory has been found so far, it is interesting to note that people who find it difficult to fall asleep tend to be deficient in, and helped by, this chemical. Sleeping pills, while helpful, do not promote deep, restful, rapid-eye-movement (REM) sleep.

According to Dr James McConnell, Professor of Psychology at the University of Michigan, REM sleep, which is associated with dreaming, may well be the key to long-term memory storage. 'Dreaming', he says, 'may be what happens as the new memory molecules go out of where they have been stored during the day. This triggers old memories, which is what we experience as dreams. That is why dreams appear to relate to what happened during the day. Other findings indicate that if you prevent REM during sleep, you have no memory.'

The synthesis of serotonin requires considerable amounts of Vitamin B_6 (pyridoxine) and it is interesting to note that a deficiency of this vitamin can be associated with lack of dreams while serotonin increases the REM portions of our sleep. (For a list of foods high in Vitamin B_6, see page 25.)

The brain makes serotonin from a common amino acid called tryptophan, which can only enter the brain by a mechanism known as active transport. It shares this mode of entry, however, with several other amino acids and so taking tryptophan may not increase brain serotonin levels unless the number of competing amino acids is also kept low.

Two ways of enhancing tryptophan's transport across the blood-brain barrier are by fasting (tryptophan should always be taken well away from meal times) or by taking some carbohydrates. The carbohydrates tend to cause the pancreas to secrete insulin which, in turn, depletes the blood stream of precisely those amino acids which are competing with tryptophan for transport across the blood-brain barrier.

While manipulating tryptophan-serotonin levels can be helpful in various conditions, it would seem that memory is worsened, if anything, by increasing tryptophan dietary intake (*New Scientist*, October, 1983, p. 47). This probably happens because the increased brain levels of serotonin, which follow the intake of tryptophan, make the brain cells more 'sleepy'.

While increased brain levels of serotonin may help some people to sleep, too much may make them unable to rest and become aggressive and suffer hallucinations. Excessive levels of serotonin

Foods containing tryptophan

alfalfa	egg
baked beans	endive
beef	fennel
beet	fish
broccoli	milk
Brussels sprouts	nuts
carrot	soya bean
cauliflower	spinach
celery	sweet potato
chicken	turkey
chive	turnip
cottage cheese	watercress

have also been associated with premature ageing and damage to the foetus. On the other hand, a deficiency of serotonin can cause depression, sleeplessness and even psychiatric disorders.

MEMORY RHYMES

Exercises to improve memory, known as mnemonics, have been known for thousands of years. The ancient Chinese used to make rhyming poems of long lists of names in order to help them remember.

Psychobiologists believe that the brain can only mark up seven separate items, or 'chunks', of information on the blackboard of short-term memory at any one time.

The ones more likely to be shifted to our permanent memory bank are those which create vivid visual images or strike a connection with something particularly eventful in our lives.

This is what mnemonic exercises are all about: a way of making otherwise boring information into something that has meaning and is interesting. A string of letters such as GTR will be remembered much more easily if we associate it with the word ALLIGATOR and make a visual image of it.

Fast thinking—glutamic acid

Fast thinking and memory go hand in hand and this requires speedy communication between brain cells. The major signaller in the human brain appears to be a simple amino acid, glutamic acid.

This chemical acts on practically every brain cell to cause rapid excitation and, in fact, it seems to be the most common 'on' signal used by sensory nerves entering the brain. This fact alone would make it the most important neurotransmitter for encoding information, that is, memory, and it may well be one of the reasons why so many researchers claim that glutamic acid appears to 'clear' the head and enhance such functions as thinking and remembering.

Another amino acid, glycine, is known to be an inhibitory transmitter at the spinal cord but the best known inhibition effect in the brain may well be that exerted by gamma-amino-butyric acid (GABA). Having a fast car with a responsive accelerator won't get you far if you are unable to slow down when you need to, so inhibitory neurotransmitters play a central role in brain functions and at least a powerful, if indirect, one in memory.

Roughly a third of all nerve cells in the brain send inhibitory rather than accelerating signals, and the chemical they use (GABA) is closely related to glutamic acid; in fact, these two are among the most common within the brain and spinal cord.

Vitamin B$_6$—too much versus too little

GABA is manufactured exclusively in the brain and spinal cord from glutamic acid and is particularly reliant on ample supplies of Vitamin B$_6$ (pyridoxine).

Glutamic acid, from which the brain makes GABA, excites while GABA itself inhibits. In a Vitamin B-deficient state, glutamic acid can reach excessive levels, causing perhaps irritability of the central nervous system. Additional intake of Vitamin B$_6$ could increase the sedating effects of GABA both by allowing more of it to be synthesised and by reducing accumulated glutamic acid.

At the same time, an excess of Vitamin B$_6$ may deplete glutamic acid reserves to the point where proper excitation, and hence perceptive functions of the nervous system, are impaired.

This may also account for the observed correlation between dreaming and Vitamin B_6 status. This correlation is one of the commonly used diagnostic methods for a naturopathic assessment of Vitamin B_6 levels in patients. Its role in memory function is peripheral at best but being unable to relax mentally could influence one's ability to memorise facts during a heavy period of studying for exams, for example.

Glutamic acid, like most amino acids, does not cross the blood-brain barrier easily so eating more foods rich in glutamic acid, or even taking it as a supplement, will have little effect. Fortunately, the brain can make its own glutamic acid from substances normally found in the diet. If the diet is low in these substances, then impaired brain function may occur.

Foods high in Vitamin B_6 (pyridoxine)

avocado	milk
barley	molasses
beans	oranges
Brazil nuts	peanuts
carrot	peas
cheese	potato
cow's milk	prunes
crab	rice
egg	soya bean
fish (cod, halibut, herring, mackerel, salmon, sardines, tuna)	spinach
	sunflower seeds
lentils	wheat bran
lima beans	wheat germ
liver (pork)	wholemeal flour
meat (beef, ham, pork)	yeast (Brewer's)

Glutamic acid can be used by the brain as fuel if and when blood-sugar levels are too low. It can also pick up and remove excessive ammonia which tends to build up during brain activity. Certainly we know that glutamic acid levels rise markedly during seizures and ammonia is also associated with ageing so that its prompt removal may help to keep brain cells younger and, therefore, smarter.

Glutamic acid has at least two other important functions. It also helps to reduce the craving for alcohol and it plays an important role in maintaining the efficiency of our immune system.

The only practical way to increase brain function with glutamic acid is by taking it in the form of L-glutamine, which is a compound that can cross to the brain and be converted to glutamic acid as required. L-glutamine has been reported to increase the IQ of mentally retarded patients.

A CASE OF POOR MENTAL FUNCTIONS AND MEMORY

Peter is a lawyer and when I first saw him he complained that his work efficiency had decreased dramatically in the past few months.

'I don't seem to be able to concentrate as well as I used to and my memory simply disappears when I most need it', he moaned. 'At first I put it down to stress, overwork—that sort of thing. I took a holiday and had a good rest. Naturally, I felt a lot better, but my brain still refused to get into gear.'

I asked Peter if he experienced his difficulties all day long or only at particular times of the day.

'In the morning, when I get to work, I am not the best and by lunchtime I can't think straight. I feel a little better after lunch but by 4 P.M. my concentration is all but gone'.

I explained to Peter that the most likely reason for his problem was that at certain times his blood-sugar levels may fall too low. This condition is called hypoglycaemia and it works in the following way. Some of the food we eat is converted into blood sugar. If the food contains a lot of sugar or consists of refined carbohydrates, like pastry or white bread, then this tends to flood the blood with sugar too quickly. The body responds to this by sending out signals which cause hormones, such as insulin, to pour out in an effort to bring the high blood-sugar level down. So, the faster and more massive the blood-sugar elevation, the greater the insulin response. And then, the blood-sugar levels drop quickly and deeply, stopping the brain from functioning efficiently. This reaction can be prevented by cutting out sugar and refined carbohydrates from the diet, and eating small and frequent

(Cont.)

Poor Mental Functions and Memory (Cont.)

snacks. There are also some supplements that can be taken to enhance brain power.

I prescribed some L-glutamine, phenylalanine, tyrosine, gingko, Vitamin B_{12} and Vitamin B_6; all nutrition factors that are involved in the formation of brain chemicals known as neurotransmitters. The 'chemicals to think by'.

I also recommended to Peter that he try several different types of breakfast and lunch foods to see which enhanced his mental powers. I explained to Peter that some of us were fast oxidisers and others were slow oxidisers: in other words, some people 'burn' carbohydrates quickly, while others do not. Therefore, it is not uncommon to find some people who function well on a breakfast of eggs, butter and wholemeal bread but can't get any energy, mental or otherwise, from breakfast cereals. At the same time, many individuals find that if they eat anything but carbohydrates in the morning, they simply feel all clogged up and tired. They do well on breakfast cereals, skimmed milk, a little jam on their toast and a cup of coffee.

Peter took my advice and, to his surprise, found that if he ate a boiled egg for breakfast and took his supplements, his brain would take off in top gear as soon as he hit the office desk. When he switched back to carbohydrates, the old symptoms would come back within a few days, although less severely because of the supplements. In addition, the tyrosine increased his ability to cope with stress and he found that phenylalanine reduced his craving for sweets.

Peter had learnt a very important lesson in nutrition: we are all biochemically different and, while general recommendations can be beneficial to most people, such as eat less fat, less sugar and more fibre, we should always try to find what is best for each one of us rather than follow generalisations.

Memory and acetylcholine

Acetylcholine is a chemical substance secreted at the ends of many nerve fibres and is responsible for transmitting nerve impulses. Acetylcholine levels in the brain are said to correlate with memory functions. Certainly conditions such as Alzheimer's disease, which produce memory loss, are associated with decreased levels of acetylcholine and we know that drugs which block the action of acetylcholine in the brain cause a temporary loss of memory function.

Unfortunately, supplementing choline (usually in the form of lecithin), which is the amino acid from which the brain makes acetylcholine, to help improve memory has failed to produce consistent results. This may, however, be due to the fact that Vitamin B_5 (pantothenic acid) and Vitamin B_1 (thiamine) are needed to convert and use choline as acetylcholine. It may well be that if these nutrients are administered in the correct amounts, together with lecithin or choline, memory enhancement could occur.

Another way to increase brain levels of acetylcholine, and a method which has been shown effective in promoting good memory, is a natural compound called deanol, introduced by Dr Carl Pfeiffer in the late 1950s. Deanol is a form of choline and appears to cross the blood-brain barrier quite easily. It is also available as DMAE (dimethyl-aminoethanol). It has been used successfully in treating memory impairment among the aged and in hyperactive children. It can also be useful in the treatment of depression, apathy and senility.

In addition to increasing acetylcholine levels, DMAE also helps the body to get rid of lipofucin, which are ageing pigments that show up as dark spots on the skin of older people and can also be found in the brains of people suffering from senility.

Foods high in choline

bean sprouts	liver (beef, pork)
beef	milk
chickpeas	peanuts
egg yolk	split peas
green beans	soya bean
lentils	

(Cont.)

(Cont.)

Foods high in Vitamin B₅ (pantothenic acid)

avocado	lobster
bean sprouts	mackerel
beef	mushrooms
chicken	peanuts
clams	pineapple
crab	salmon
egg	sardines
haddock	soya bean
lentils	watermelon
liver (beef, pork)	wheat germ

Foods high in Vitamin B₁ (thiamine)

beef (heart, liver, kidney)	pork (liver)
Brazil nuts	poultry
cereals	pumpkin
fish (mackerel, perch, red snapper)	soya bean
	sunflower seeds
lamb	wheat
milk	wheat germ
oatmeal	yeast (Brewer's)
peas and other legumes	

Learning and RNA

Ribonucleic acid (RNA), a basic structure of the blueprint for life, appears to be essential for learning processes. Several alleged memory enhancers, such as orotic acid, are in fact converted to RNA. Orotic acid is a substance found in milk. Orotate combined with minerals such as magnesium, potassium or calcium are available as supplements in health food stores. High doses of RNA are needed to produce memory enhancement but there is the added advantage that RNA helps cell protection against oxidising agents which cause cellular ageing. Unfortunately, RNA does have some drawbacks:

- Its acidity can cause stomach upsets.
- RNA metabolism produces large amounts of uric acid which can cause, or aggravate, gout and also precipitate into crystals which can deposit in the joints and kidneys.

Shopping for memory enhancers is like shopping for anything else: learn the facts or you will waste money. Some health food stores carry RNA but unless a product contains more than 12 per cent it is probably just yeast. Yeast contains about 6 per cent RNA, but hardly any of it is available to the body as it is behind cell walls that we cannot break down. The body, of course, makes RNA and one way to stimulate RNA synthesis is to take Vitamin B_{12}.

The adrenaline connection and memory enhancers

Norepinephrine, a chemical cousin of adrenaline (epinephrine), is another neurotransmitter which plays an important role in moods and behaviour, and may well be associated with memory. Its synthesis begins with the amino acid tyrosine which is converted to dopamine. Excessive amounts of dopamine, which is a neurotransmitter in its own right, are associated with schizophrenia.

We know that amphetamines can cause psychosis and we also know that amphetamines are triggers for the release of brain dopamine. In fact, some of the most successful anti-psychotic drugs work by binding the dopamine receptors in the brain and therefore preventing their activation by the transmitter. Vitamin C (ascorbic acid) and Vitamin B_3 (niacinamide) are also said to have the same effect.

The principal dopamine enzyme, dopamine beta hydroxylase, is both calcium and Vitamin-C dependent which probably accounts for the observed calming effects of these nutrients. Dopamine is eventually converted to norepinephrine which also plays a very important role in the control of human behaviour and moods. Low levels of norepinephrine are closely associated with depression and an inability to think clearly.

WHY COFFEE IS A STIMULANT

Most people know that caffeine and theophylline (active ingredients of coffee and tea) can help you to 'wake up'. Coffee is a 'natural' substance which belongs to a chemical group known as methylxanthines.

Methylxanthines inhibit the enzyme (phosphodiesterase) which destroys cyclic adenosine monophosphate (cAMP), the principal activator of most, if not all, neurotransmitters in the brain. So anything which tends to lower phosphodiesterase levels will enhance neurotransmitter activities, and that is exactly what caffeine does.

Vitamin C (ascorbic acid) acts in the same way: it inhibits phosphodiesterase and increases cAMP levels in the brain. If it weren't for the fact that a cup of Vitamin C can also cause diarrhoea, we could easily substitute it for our morning coffee.

In spite of this, most orthodox psychiatrists continue to say that caffeine stimulates the brain but deny that Vitamin C has any effect whatsoever, apart from preventing scurvy. So whether you fancy coffee or a cup of Vitamin C, you can rest assured that it will help your brain to function a little better—for a while at least.

Adrenaline

Adrenaline (epinephrine) is the adrenal counterpart of the brain's own norepinephrine and is one of the most significant memory enhancers our body makes.

People learn best when they are motivated, alert and stimulated. During the Second World War German pilots were able to fly non-stop at night from Germany to England. This was no mean feat in those days and it demanded superhuman powers of concentration. A captured Luftwaffe pilot was found to have been injected with an extract of a brain chemical known to stimulate the adrenal glands (which largely control how alert we are).

Research centres in the United States worked to reproduce this substance, adrenocortical stimulating hormone (ACTH), which stimulates the production and release of natural steroids. It also became clear that when the adrenal glands produce epinephrine (adrenaline), mnemonic abilities were enhanced significantly.

In the late 1970s, a brilliant series of experiments by James McGaugh, Professor of Psychobiology at the University of California, showed clearly that the brain's ability to memorise can be influenced by drugs that affect the levels of both epinephrine (adrenaline) and norepinephrine (noradrenaline).

Foods containing phenylalanine

almonds	egg
apple	fish (herring)
avocado	milk
baked beans	parsley
banana	peanuts
beef	pineapple
beet	soya bean
carrot	soy proteins
chicken	spinach
cottage cheese	tomato
chocolate	

Foods containing tyrosine

alfalfa	carrot
almonds	cheese
apple	cherries
apricot	chicken
asparagus	chocolate
avocado	cottage cheese
baked beans	cucumber
banana	egg
beef	fig
beet	fish (herring)
capsicum	leek

(Cont.)

Food containing tyrosine (Cont.)

lettuce	soy proteins
milk	spinach
parsley	strawberries
peanuts	watercress
poultry	watermelon
soya bean	yoghurt

Although only small amounts of these chemicals are found in the brain, the large amounts secreted by the adrenals during a state of excitement appear to be the primary factor in memory. Because adrenal secretions are the primary responses of the body to stress stimuli, it would seem that strong emotions act, as it were, as an embalming fluid for memories. It is almost as if an event will not become part of our conscious experience unless adrenal hormones cry out 'print it!' If emotions and chemicals are the 'ink' of memory, then the complex circuitry of nerve cells and their myriad connections are the 'paper' on which events are recorded.

FOODS TO THINK BY

Foods, drugs and several beverages have always been associated with creativity in one way or another.

Alcohol and fermented beverages have played a prominent role in the creative process for writers, notably Hemingway, Faulkner and Fitzgerald, who all used alcohol extensively to enhance their creative moods.

Faulkner once said he couldn't even begin to write without a bottle of Scotch nearby, while the famous mathematician Poincaré found coffee essential to his work and Housman, the English poet, found that beer and tea were essential to his work.

Chocolate can also be a powerful stimulant, probably because the brain uses one of its chemicals, phenylethylalanine, to manufacture norepinephrine.

(Cont.)

Foods to Think By (Cont.)

An unusual chemical called thujione, which is related to nutmeg, is said to exert a powerful stimulating effect on the brain. A constituent of absinthe, this chemical is added in small quantities to vermouth and is a major component of cedar leaf oil.

Irrespective of what you may need to think better, one thing seems clear: large meals make thinking more difficult while fasting enhances the creative processes.

Phenylalanine is a precursor, or source, of norepinephrine and this amino acid can be found in meat, cheese and chocolate. It is also available as an amino acid supplement and is an excellent natural painkiller, antidepressant and memory enhancer. Its only drawbacks are that it is very expensive and may elevate blood pressure in sensitive people. When used properly, it is probably the best natural antidepressant available today.

Tyrosine is another amino acid that produces norepinephrine. Levels of tyrosine in the brain are reliant on dietary levels of tyrosine, Vitamin B_{12} and magnesium.

The neuropeptides

The discovery of chemical signal modulators, the neuropeptides (small protein fragments), has caused a flurry of activity among neurobiologists as they try to clarify their role in brain functions. Neuropeptides seem, at this stage, to have a dual role. They are capable of triggering off complex behavioural responses when applied to the brain, and in most other parts of the body they act as local hormones, or regulators.

Vasopressin, a neuropeptide and an antidiuretic hormone produced by the pituitary gland, can increase memory when applied to the brain. A synthetic form of vasopressin found in nasal sprays has been reported to restore memory to amnesia patients and to improve concentration ('Mind Foods', *Omni*, Jan. 1983, p. 40).

At this point in time, the biological significance of using the same chemical for apparently quite different purposes is not clear but the field is one that promises many surprises.

INCREASING YOUR BRAIN POWER

Many nutritional scientists have found that some vitamins enhance brain function. I have often seen an improvement of mental ability occur as the result of treatment which involved the use of vitamins for other problems.

Brain cells, like all body cells, need to be constantly supplied with molecules derived from the nutrients in the food you eat in order to function properly. Because the brain cells' functions involve thinking, anything that results in less than optimal nutrition for the brain cells will result in less than optimal thinking by the brain.

- It has been discovered that **Vitamin C** interacts with an enzyme called phosphodiesterase which reduces the brain levels of cyclic AMP, and therefore raises all brain cell responses to normal. Vitamin C is abundant in peppers, capsicums, tomatoes and citrus fruits.
- It has also been found that **choline** or **lecithin** is essential for proper brain cell communication, attention span and motor co-ordination. This substance has also been associated with improved mental ability. Choline, or lecithin, is found in whole grains, beans (particularly soya beans), cold pressed oils such as sunflower, safflower and sesame; and lecithin granules and capsules.
- **Vitamin B$_5$** (pantothenic acid) has been found to help children with learning difficulties.
- **Vitamin B$_6$** (pyridoxine) is essentially linked with the formation of several important brain chemicals and the integrity of the nervous system. This vitamin has been reported to produce mental improvement in children suffering from a variety of problems ranging from autism to hyperactivity.
- **Copper** tends to over-excite brain cells. **Zinc** is capable of counteracting the action of copper in the body and therefore minimises its nasty effects on the brain.
- **Zinc** deficiencies have been linked with autism.
- Low levels of vitamins have been linked, in general, with excess activity of the nervous system and an inability to concentrate.

(Cont.)

Increasing Your Brain Power (Cont.)

- Gamma aminobutyric acid (GABA) helps cells in different parts of the brain to communicate with each other. This is made in the brain from glutamic acid, which is an ordinary amino acid present in food. This conversion, however, is only possible with the help of Vitamin B_6.
- Glutamic acid also picks up excessive ammonia from the brain cells. A form of glutamic acid called L-glutamine is particularly effective in this function and it has been shown to improve thinking, clear the brains of alcoholics, reduce foggy minds during hangovers and improve early morning alertness.
- Norepinephrine, another brain neurotransmitter which is associated with brain alertness, is derived from the amino acids **tyrosine** and **phenylalanine**. Brain levels of norepinephrine are related to the dietary levels of tyrosine, Vitamin B_{12} and magnesium.
- Ribonucleic acid (**RNA**) is now believed to be the stuff of which memory is made. RNA is plentiful in eggs, fish and other high-protein foods. However, the body needs Vitamin B_6 to break down the proteins into amino acids and Vitamin B_{12} and inositol to make RNA.
- Reduced thinking ability can be the effect of peroxidation and free radicals. **Vitamin E**, **Vitamin A**, **carotene** and **Vitamin C** help to protect brain cells against this.
- Antioxidants also help against free radicals. There are several amino acids and nutrients that are important: para amino benzoic acid (PABA), L-cysteine, taurine, gingko, magnesium, zinc, ginseng, garlic, methionine and selenium.
- The metabolic rate of the whole body is regulated by a gland called the thyroid. The functions of this gland are enhanced by kelp and iodine.

2

MOOD SWINGS—HOW TO CONTROL THEM

Moods are very subjective. What may be considered a neurotic outburst by one person, may be a show of normal temperament by another. However, the inability to keep an emotional even keel in the face of life's daily waves and the constant switch between anger and love, hyperactivity and depression can reach dramatic proportions in some individuals.

There are many reasons for having uncontrollable mood swings: some reasons are simple and obvious and others are obscure and very, very complex. So, let us look at some of the possible causes for up-and-down moods and then look at some of the ways to control them without the use of drugs.

How histamine affects your moods

Histapenia and histadelia refer to a condition in which there is either too much or too little histamine in the brain. Both conditions can alter the way we behave. The body has two separate receptors for histamine: H_1 which is involved in the classic histamine allergic reactions, such as headaches, and H_2, which is a brain receptor.

Excessive histamine levels

People with excessive histamine levels (histadelics) have a large capacity for alcohol and other drugs. They tend to have a high libido (sex drive) and are subjected to periodic and deep bouts of depression. Although their bouts of depression may be short and relatively infrequent, when they do occur this type of person may well entertain suicidal thoughts. They seem to need less sleep than most people and tend to be somewhat obsessive, but are strangely sensitive to physical pain. They often suffer low or fluctuating blood-sugar levels (hypoglycaemia) and adrenal exhaustion (hypoadrenocorticism) because they tend to be fast metabolisers. These conditions appear to fluctuate widely, from week to week and even from day to day. They tend to have some allergies or intolerances which are often well masked, and they are prone to headaches or migraines. Good teeth and bad stomachs are two more signs. The teeth are good because histadelics salivate a lot and stomach ulcers occur because they are tense.

Blood tests can be used to determine histamine levels. A request for a differential white cell count will indicate a basophil count. Normal range for basophils is somewhere between 10 and 140. A high figure indicates high histamine levels.

Other common tests used to indicate histamine levels are the mean corpuscular volume (MCV) and the mean corpuscular haemoglobin content (MCHC). The MCV measures how large red blood cells are, and MCHC measures how much haemoglobin they contain. A low MCV and a high MCHC points to the possibility of high histamine levels.

Treatment

The main thrust of orthomolecular treatment is aimed at reducing histamine levels. Methionine, an essential amino acid, tends to methylate histamine and deactivate it. Pangamic acid, also known as calcium pangamate or Vitamin B_{15}, is also useful in reducing histamine levels, as is a diet high in cabbages, especially the Chinese red variety.

Vitamin C has a natural antihistamine effect, while calcium tends to help the release of histamine.

Pharmaceutical drugs such as Dilantin® (only available by prescription) can be used, as these interfere with Vitamin B_{12} and folic acid metabolism (Vitamin B_{12} enhances the production of histamine). However, natural therapists prefer not to use drugs, although it is sometimes necessary to bring about fast results. In this case, the drug should only be used for a couple of weeks, gradually reduced and then eventually withdrawn after a month or so.

Taking large amounts of supplements, such as tyrosine, phenylalanine or pantothenic acid may, however, be counterproductive as they tend to stimulate the nervous system which is already over-stimulated by the excessive histamine.

A thorough check for food intolerances/allergies is mandatory and fasting will generally help, since histamine synthesis is slowed down by a lack of proteins.

Foods containing methionine

apple	garlic
beef	ham
Brazil nuts	liver
Brussels sprouts	milk
cabbage	pineapple
cauliflower	pork
chicken	sardines
chives	soy
cottage cheese	soya bean
egg	watercress
fish	yoghurt

Foods high in Vitamin B_{15} (pangamic acid)

almonds	rice bran
apricot kernels	rice shoots
liver	yeast (Brewer's)

Low histamine levels

Histapenics are people who suffer from a deficiency of the neuro-transmitter histamine which causes fluctuating moods. Their mean corpuscular volume tends to be high, pointing to a deficiency of dietary or absorbed Vitamin B_{12} and folic acid. A routine blood test will often also show a low basophil count (usually well below 10).

Although they appear to have rapid mood swings, the tendency is usually on the down side. They are likely to be day-dreamers, often out of touch with reality and, generally speaking, they are low achievers who show little productivity in their work or chosen career. They are easily frustrated and become quite irritable and, as soon as they are under stress, they become physically tired and easily depressed. They get drunk on very small amounts of alcohol and are easily affected by most drugs. They generally seem to need a lot of sleep. They have a lowish sex drive and a slow metabolism and can generally tolerate pain quite easily. There appears to be a touch of paranoia in their makeup (thinking the world is against them).

Treatment

Treatment for histapenics involves large doses of Vitamin B_{12} to increase histamine levels. Large doses can be given by injections or taken orally. Injections of Vitamin B_{12} can cause problems with people who are allergic or hypersensitive to yeast and so care should be taken with this treatment. Vitamin B_{12} taken orally seldom produces any problems. Vitamin B_{12} Plus tablets have been found to be very effective.

Folic acid, however, does seem to increase the effects of oestrogen and it may be contraindicated in some patients with the following history: mammary tumours; hyperoestrogenism; and a type of premenstrual syndrome which is characterised by excessive menstrual blood (menorrhagia) which is often clotty, breast swelling and tenderness, lethargy rather than irritability during the premenstrual phase and a tendency to retain a great deal of fluid (see chapter on Premenstrual syndrome).

More recent research also indicates that people with the above history should not take yeast supplements as they may be allergic to yeast or have a yeast infection, which may make the problem worse.

Foods high in Vitamin B₁₂ (cyanocobalamine)

beef (kidney, liver)	pork (hearts, liver)
cheese (cheddar, cream)	prunes
chicken	salmon
egg yolk	sardines
herring	shellfish
mackerel	tuna
milk	yoghurt

Foods high in folic acid

almonds	orange
asparagus	peanuts
avocado	pecans
barley	plums
beef (heart, liver)	raisins
blackberries	rice
cottage cheese	spinach
dates	tuna
legumes	turkey
lettuce	walnuts
Lima beans	wheat germ
mackerel	

Unless they are intolerant or allergic to buckwheat, this food is a valuable source of rutin, which prevents the breakdown of histidine. (Rutin can be taken in tablet form.)

Niacin, not niacinamide, should be given to help the conversion of histidine to histamine and a thorough check for wheat, gluten and grain sensitivity should be made by a food provocation test. Other tests for detecting food sensitivities are not as reliable as the food provocation test. RAST tests only measure immunoglobin E reactions and most food allergies are mediated by other immunoglobins. The cytotoxic test is very old and has proven to be unreliable and not reproducible. More up-to-date tests, such as the

ALCAT test, are now available; however, they can be very costly and are inferior to the food provocation test.

Phenylalanine, tryptophan and tyrosine may be helpful as depression is often connected with a deficiency of these neurotransmitters. My clinical experience has been that tryptophan can worsen the symptoms of some psychiatric patients. If the underlying problem is a lack of norepinephrine, increasing serotonin (the product of tryptophan) will cause further imbalances of the ratio between the two neurotransmitters (serotonin from tryptophan and norepinephrine from tyrosine). If, however, the underlying problem is a deficiency of serotonin, tryptophan may be used successfully.

Vitamin B_5, or pantothenic acid, can also be a useful supplement because of its role in the transmission of nerve impulses in the brain and in helping the adrenal glands respond to stress.

Foods high in niacin

avocado	potato
baked beans	raspberries
barley	rice
beef	salmon
broccoli	soy proteins
chicken	squash
clams	strawberries
fish (haddock, halibut)	tomato
liver	tuna
mushrooms	turkey
organ meats (liver, kidney)	watermelon
oysters	wheat
peanuts	yeast (Brewer's)
pork	

In all cases, whether high or low histamine levels are suspected, a tissue saturation test for Vitamin C should be performed in addition to the routine urine analysis carried out during the food allergy test.

Anxiety (LIAS) and agoraphobia

THE CASE OF JOANNA X

Joanna, a thirty-year-old business executive who travels all over the world as part of her job came to see me some time ago.

'To put it quite bluntly, Dr Vayda,' she said, 'I think I am about to get the sack. I am very good at my job and was promoted relatively early to a top buyer position about a year ago. After a few months of travelling, I began to experience episodes of what I call a "foggy brain" and anxiety. All of a sudden, and for no apparent reason, I would just be unable to think. Things that I would normally do almost without even thinking would be totally forgotten or, quite abruptly, I would find myself almost incapable of carrying out the simplest task. I could not add up or make a decision about a particular line or even think coherently about what I was supposed to do. After a few such episodes, I began to feel fearful and often panicky—for no apparent reason.

'I would spend hours on end shaking and feeling something terrible was going to happen to me. I began to be afraid of leaving the hotel room—the only place, I may add, where I felt safe. I knew the feeling was somewhat similar to those I heard described as agoraphobia.

'I was not sick, yet I felt unwell. I didn't have a cold, or a temperature or the flu; yet parts of my body began to ache in a subtle but disconcerting way. A number of doctors put me through every imaginable test but could only tell me I was perfectly healthy. I was told over and over again that it was all in my mind or the stress of my job. Jet lag, premenstrual syndrome were blamed, as was the fact that I was unmarried, worked too hard or did not have any children. It really boiled down to the particular personal beliefs of the attending physician. Yet in my own heart I *knew* something else was wrong. Although it clearly affected my brain, I also knew I was not mad, or neurotic.

'I took a week off in Honolulu, sat on the beach, swam, sunbathed and generally rested. I did not improve much although I felt less

(Cont.)

The Case of Joanna X (Cont.)

anxious. So much for the suggestion that I just needed a holiday. And anyway, I had only been working for a couple of months since my last break; hardly the stuff to put a healthy thirty-year-old out of action. By the end of the week I convinced myself there was nothing I could do about it and went back to work. I am afraid that, unless I can find a way to calm down, I will have to take tranquillisers or risk getting the sack.'

I asked Joanna if she participated in any sport and she told me that she usually played some tennis but since being unwell she found she lacked the energy. 'Anyway,' she added, almost as an after-thought, 'whenever I exert myself physically I feel the symptoms either begin or, if already present, get worse, particularly the anxiety.' For me this last statement clinched the diagnosis.

A short series of questions established that Joanna drank moder-ately, but daily, at least with her meals, and that she drank about 4 or 5 cups of coffee and perhaps 2 cups of tea each day. Her diet included a fair amount of sweets and often she resorted to fast-food snacks which consisted primarily of refined carbohydrates. Her med-ical history revealed the fact that she had suffered a bout of hepatitis a few years previously.

I reassured Joanna that she was not likely to be allergic to any-thing and that allergies had nothing to do with her condition. Joanna was not mentally ill either. Although she did exhibit and experience the symptoms of anxiety neurosis, Joanna did not need to take a sin-gle tranquilliser. However, within a few months she was back to her normal self. You see, Joanna was suffering from lactate induced anx-iety syndrome (LIAS), a condition that may be responsible for between 20 and 50 per cent of all anxiety cases.

Joanna's impaired liver was not able to perform some of the key steps in the biochemical chain which breaks down carbohydrates into glucose. She produced, instead, abnormal amounts of a form of lactic acid called lactate. This natural chemical is a known panico-genic, which means it is capable of causing anxiety, or panic, in sus-ceptible individuals.

Foods high in Vitamin B$_5$ (pantothenic acid)

avocado	lobster
bean sprouts	mackerel
beef	mushrooms
chicken	peanuts
clams	pineapple
crab	salmon
egg	sardines
haddock	soya bean
lentils	watermelon
liver (beef, pork)	wheat germ

Anxiety has different meanings for many people: irritable, nervous, fearful, panicky, touchy, excitable, moody, terrified, apprehensive. These are all words commonly used to describe a state of mind which makes some people afraid to confront or cope with everyday tasks. Some people begin to sweat profusely at the thought of going out for a job interview, or meeting a new person, while others cannot even bear to get on a bus or go down to the corner shop. (In extreme cases, this condition is known as agoraphobia.)

One symptom which is common in almost all types of anxiety is a constant, or cyclic, lack of energy. Other signs include: a rapid heart beat, palpitations, a feeling of inner shakiness (often accompanied by actual physical and visible shaking of the hands, limbs or even the whole body), a feeling of tightness in the throat, muscular cramps and moist palms.

Many sufferers experience mental confusion, unsteadiness, even dizziness, plus intermittent feelings of extreme fear and hopelessness accompanied by a sense of impending doom. It is very common indeed for such people to be labelled 'neurotic' by friends, relatives and sometimes even their own doctor.

On physical examination, someone suffering from anxiety will have elevated diastolic blood pressure; however, in cases where tiredness is a major symptom, blood pressure may be quite low. There is a tendency towards muscular cramps and heart rates tend to be abnormally fast. Invariably, people suffering from anxiety find it difficult to sleep and tire easily.

While some may have a history of psychiatric illness, many more have been classified as 'neurotic' and a fair proportion of them have a history of alcohol abuse, liver disorders, mal-absorption and recurrent thrush, low or fluctuating blood-sugar levels (hypoglycaemia) and environmental and food hypersensitivities or allergies. Breathing disorders are also common. Some studies have shown that most, if not all, such patients derive up to 75 per cent of their calories from refined carbohydrates and sugars.

In many cases the patient will report a worsening of symptoms immediately after strenuous physical effort. They describe themselves, and are often referred to, as people who 'live on their nerves'. Paradoxically, this kind of individual often has an overwhelming need for solitude and a lack of sensory inputs.

While it is true that in some cases of anxiety neurosis or agoraphobia the patient has an underlying personality disorder or psychological problem, there are many instances where the syndrome is due to biochemical abnormalities that are related to nutritional imbalances or deficiencies.

One of the most common nutritional imbalances is an excess of lactate. Lactate is the ionic form of lactic acid—a normal by-product of metabolism—which increases during physical activity and muscular exertion. Lactate can trigger a panic or anxiety attack and, if too much lactate is present in the blood all the time, the patient may well be in a constant state of anxiety.

Experiments have shown that in more than 90 per cent of anxious people and some 20 per cent of 'normal' individuals an intravenous injection of lactate will cause an immediate anxiety attack. Normally some of the circulating lactate is broken down to carbon dioxide and water and expelled from the body. An individual's capacity to break down lactate varies and there are many reasons for an excessive build-up of lactate in the blood stream.

Digested starches, sugars, refined carbohydrates, and honey sorbitol or fructose (fruit sugar) are converted to glucose (blood sugar) in several biochemical steps. In one of these steps, pyruvate is formed and too much of this may be converted to lactate when the liver is not functioning very well, or when there is a deficiency in some of the B-group vitamins (notably Vitamin B_1 (thiamine),

Vitamin B_3 (niacin) and Vitamin B_6 (pyridoxine)) and minerals such as magnesium or zinc.

Pyruvate is also associated with Vitamin B_{12} and a deficiency of Vitamin B_{12} can cause pyruvate levels to increase dramatically. Increased pyruvate levels can cause blood-sugar levels to plummet and the resulting hypoglycaemia causes its own set of secondary symptoms, such as lethargy and mental confusion.

An interesting property of lactate is that it forms a bond with circulating calcium. It is this property that has led to the use of calcium supplements in the treatment of anxiety. Calcium binds excess lactate in the bloodstream and therefore reduces the possibility of a lactate-induced anxiety attack. Calcium supplements are not used to cure anxiety neurosis or agoraphobia but to prevent, or avoid, anxiety attacks altogether.

Another approach to treating anxiety is aimed at increasing liver function with the correct diet (often moderately high in proteins and sometimes high in fibre) and supplements. Vitamin C powder is used in the form of calcium ascorbate partly because ascorbic acid increases the synthesis of cyclic AMP (which stimulates the liver's uptake of lactate) and because the calcium will also tie up some of the excess lactate.

We never use bone meal because of possible heavy-metal toxicity, or calcium gluconate because it is poorly absorbed. Calcium lactate is not used because the calcium and lactate neutralise each other and there is insufficient 'free' calcium to latch onto circulating lactate.

Calcium needs to be taken on an empty stomach at least two hours after a meal or one hour before. Tea, coffee and other caffeine-containing preparations are not advised because they can increase the lactate-pyruvate ratio. Alcohol also has a similar effect and, in addition, it can jeopardise optimal liver functions. Drastic reduction in the consumption of fruit juices, honey and other sources of fructose are recommended as this sugar is quickly converted to lactate under anaerobic conditions.

A low-sugar, no-refined-carbohydrates diet, similar to the hypo-glycaemic regimen, is suggested for people suffering with LIAS and the patient is advised to sweat profusely (preferably in a sauna and not through exercise), because sweating is one way in which the body can rid itself of lactate.

Foods high in calcium

almonds	molasses
Brazil nuts	oysters
broccoli	salmon
cheese (cottage)	sardines
clams	sesame seeds
crab	soya bean
egg yolk	turnip greens
legumes	vegetables (dark green,
liver (beef, chicken)	leafy ones)
mackerel	yoghurt
milk	

After a trial period, the patient is reassessed for each specific symptom and, if any of them persist, each one is looked at again for the possibility of a different cause.

Hypoglycaemia

Hypoglycaemia is fluctuating blood sugar where the levels either drop to an abnormally low level or fluctuate widely or rapidly. It is one of the most common causes of erratic behaviour, especially if it causes unexplained fatigue, occasional dizziness and a craving for sweets.

While no longer considered a 'disease' in itself, hypoglycaemia is often associated with a junk-food diet that contains too many sugars. It can be triggered off by white, brown, raw or crystal sugar as quickly as it can be triggered off by honey and molasses. In fact, refined carbohydrates, cakes, soft drinks and even an excessive amount of dried fruit can cause the symptoms.

The underlying cause of this condition, which is really a symptom, is often an intolerance, hypersensitivity or allergy to a common food, chemical or environmental factor. In women at least, another very common cause can be candida infestation, commonly known as thrush or monilia.

In the old days we used to carry out a glucose tolerance test (GTT) over a period of several hours for diagnosis. Nowadays, the test is still carried out, but instead of sugar, different foods or chemicals are used to challenge the patient, while several different parameters are measured along with the fluctuations in blood-sugar levels.

Irrespective of the cause of hypoglycaemia, we know that it can invariably be triggered off by sugar, so the basis of the old hypoglycaemic diet (no sugar or sweets or refined carbohydrates plus small but frequent snacks) is still used. The actual foods in the diet, however, depend on the individual's susceptibility. Some people may still be placed on a high-protein diet while others may be on a high-fibre diet and others still on special regimens which eliminate particular foods.

Vitamins and mineral supplements are always tailored to the individual. If the hypoglycaemic is depressed most of the time, Vitamin B_5 will help a lot. If there is a great deal of anxiety and irritability, it may make things worse. Zinc, Vitamin B, Vitamin C (in this case not calcium ascorbate) and other supplements are also given.

Foods high in Vitamin B_5 (pantothenic acid)

avocado	lobster
bean sprouts	mackerel
beef	mushrooms
chicken	peanuts
clams	pineapple
crab	salmon
eggs	sardines
haddock	soya bean
lentils	watermelon
liver (beef, pork)	wheat germ

Foods high in zinc

bran	mushrooms
Brazil nuts	oatmeal
crab	oysters
egg	pork
grains	pumpkin seeds
herring	rice, brown
kidney	sunflower seeds
lamb	tuna
liver (beef)	veal
milk	yeast (Brewer's)

Foods high in Vitamin C (ascorbic acid)

alfalfa	citrus fruit (lemons, oranges, tomatoes)
banana	guava
berries (blueberries, gooseberries, raspberries and strawberries)	kidney
Brazil nuts	liver (beef)
broccoli	oysters
Brussels sprouts	potato
cabbage	spinach
cantaloupe melon	sweet potato
capsicum	vegetables (green leafy ones)
cauliflower	watermelon

Because the liver is intimately involved in the storing of blood sugar, it is essential that liver functions are maximised with an appropriate diet and supplements and that total abstinence from alcohol is maintained.

Medical drugs which affect the liver should only be used if absolutely necessary and with the utmost care. Because stress influences both our immune system and our sugar metabolism, relaxation, meditation, and removing stressful situations, are recommended.

WHAT HAPPENS WHEN YOU DEVELOP AN ALLERGY?

Your body develops antibodies against the offending food or substance, and forever after, when antibody and allergen meet, a small
explosion occurs in your body and various chemical substances (like
histamine) are released. Your body aims to fight what it sees as the
enemy but, in the process, body tissues can become irritated or
injured.

   If the tissues, which are made up of cells, happen to be in the lining of your air passages, you sneeze, cough or develop sinusitis; if
they are in the intestinal passages, your digestion suffers; if brain
cells are thus affected, you develop psychiatric symptoms. Allergies
are very problematic because you never know which guise they'll
take and which part of the body will be the innocent bystander that
gets knocked down in the scuffle between antigen and allergen.

Allergies and candida (thrush)

Allergies and candida are intimately interwoven and, apart from
causing the hypoglycaemic syndrome, they can also be responsible
for unbelievable mood swings. I have seen and treated thousands of
patients whose emotional life has been restored to reasonable levels
simply by detecting and then treating their unsuspected intolerances, allergies or hypersensitivities. With candida, the problem is
far more complicated.

Candida infection is usually only noticed if and when it affects the
vaginal, oral or nail area. Vaginal candidiasis, to give it a medical name,
causes a strong itch, sometimes a smelly discharge and uncomfortable
sexual intercourse.

Candida, the yeast fungus responsible for candidiasis, inhabits the
mouth, throat, intestine and genito-urinary tract of most humans. It
normally causes no problem and is, as it were, a 'silent partner'.
When our natural resistance is compromised, it begins to proliferate
and take over. Any weakening of the immune system by stress, poor
diet, sickness or the use of certain drugs can cause a candida overgrowth.

Candidiasis cannot usually be diagnosed by orthodox methods, so a thorough medical and nutritional history is essential. Candida overgrowth invariably causes a sensitivity (intolerance or allergy, if you like) to yeast and other moulds or fungi and one of the most common mistakes made by well-meaning practitioners is to treat the condition without diagnosing and correcting the multiple allergies which are invariably present.

Symptoms and signs include premenstrual syndrome; a craving for sweets, bread, cakes, fermented, smoked or pickled foods;

WHY ARE ALLERGIES MORE PREVALENT NOWADAYS?

1. More and more of us survive birth.
2. More and more of us are not breast fed, and therefore miss the colostrum which helps to build the immune system.
3. More and more of us eat a diet which is up to 50 per cent manufactured, processed and synthesised and it is from an increasingly narrower range of ingredients. Both these factors are prime ways to encourage allergies. A survey conducted in 2003 found that families across the UK are eating more ready-cooked and takeaway meals than ever before. It is estimated that a staggering £1,430 million a year is spent on takeaway meals in Britain.
4. More and more of our food contains substances that people cannot handle, such as wheat, sugar and caffeine.
5. More and more pollutants are bobbing up in everything from your favourite aftershave to the fertiliser used to grow your vegetables. And city water may contain up to 200 chemicals!
6. More and more materials we place next to our body, or put up in the house, are, in fact, by-products of petrochemical hydrocarbons which are highly allergenic substances. So our homes, offices, cars and shops contain more and more potential allergens.

To reduce your chances of becoming susceptible to many of the allergens around, try to avoid synthetic materials, denatured, processed foods and chemical contaminants, and try to live the natural life as much as you can.

abdominal distension; colitis; constipation; diarrhoea; flatulence; headaches; depression; irritability; anxiety; sinusitis; asthma; cystitis; fatigue; joint pains or stiffness; fluid retention; skin problems; and an inability to lose weight despite many strict diets.

As the organism continues to grow, it changes from its normal yeast-fungal form, in which it causes the hypersensitivity and allergy, to a mycelial-fungal form, which produces rhizoids. Rhizoids are long, root-like structures which are able to penetrate the gut wall and break down the normal barriers between the intestine and the blood.

Because of the breakdown in the barriers, many compounds enter the circulation and cause allergic reactions. If these compounds penetrate the blood-brain barrier, they can produce symptoms which can be very easily mistaken for mental illness. These incompletely digested proteins (polypeptides) have even been known to mimic 'real' neurotransmitters and play havoc with our moods.

Candidiasis, and its far ranging systemic effects, needs to be carefully treated by an experienced orthomolecular practitioner. Firstly the candida organism must be destroyed. This is only achieved with an antifungal preparation (nystatin) which must be carefully administered. At the same time, the organism is literally starved with a diet that is yeast-free and has no refined carbohydrates and sugars. The immunological resistance of each patient must be restored with a combination of supplements and ecological care.

Even when this has been achieved, and it can take anything from a few weeks to many months, the patient must be carefully monitored (via challenge tests) for any residual allergies. Then a variety of probiotics, such as lactobacillus acidophilus, should be used to foster the growth of bacteria in the gut that normally keep the candida organisms at bay.

Even after successful elimination of excessive candida, the intestinal mucosa should be restored with a diet high in fibre, oleic acid and biotin (a B-group vitamin which is available in egg yolk and liver). If this type of diet is not possible because of a grain allergy, glucomannan is used instead. After this phase, several specially formulated supplements are used to help restore the intestinal mucosa. Garlic is often used in conjunction with these measures.

Unfortunately, after treating many hundreds of patients with olive oil, biotin and a high-fibre diet, we have found that it does not work very often. The man who first proposed this programme, Dr J. Bland says: 'Although not entirely successful, this programme has been helpful . . . employed to alleviate symptoms of chronic conditions.' It is effective in chronic states, but it seldom seems to cure the underlying condition. While the changes to mycelial candida are slowed down, the excessive growth of fungal candida sets up a powerful intolerance and saps the immuno-competence of the host.

A CASE OF CANDIDA ALLERGY

Melissa was plagued by recurrent ear infection, skin rashes and sinusitis. She was experiencing terrible mood swings and severe premenstrual syndrome symptoms, especially depression. She had also had thrush a few times in the past five years.

Her doctor, a general practitioner with an interest in nutrition and alternative medicine, had diagnosed candidiasis and prescribed antifungals as well as a yeast-free diet. Melissa felt quite terrible after taking the medicine but her doctor explained to her that this was probably a 'die-off' reaction which would last only a few days while her body killed off the offending organisms. Unfortunately, the symptoms persisted and she was forced to abandon the treatment.

I explained to Melissa that this was not at all uncommon, as many of these so-called die-off reactions were, in fact, an 'allergic' reaction to candida. The clue was that the symptoms persisted after the four or five days during which a die-off is likely to occur. In fact, a die-off reaction is often diagnostic evidence of fungi and mould allergies. I also explained to Melissa that treatment for a candida infection is quite different from that for a candida allergy.

Candida infections usually require the concurrent treatment of one's sex partner and often of any other individuals, such as children, who come in daily and close contact with the sufferer.

Candida can cause infections as well as allergies: allergies are caused by altering the immune system and infections are caused by the release of toxins. Candida can cause both in any one individual. Such a situation can result in a variety of symptoms which involve

(Cont.)

A Case of Candida Allergy (Cont.)

organs and glands anywhere in the body—even those remote from the areas infected by the organism. Candidiasis can be associated with foods, chemicals, environmental allergies or intolerances or sensitivities as well as dysfunctions of many glands and, therefore, hormone and enzyme systems.

The symptoms of allergy to candida are similar to those of allergies or intolerances to moulds and fungi, with one exception: the so-called 'die-off' reaction can last a lot longer and be so severe as to impede treatment if an infection is present at the same time. Let me explain: sometimes when treatment with antifungal begins, dying candida organisms are re-absorbed and, because they change and release toxins, this causes a worsening of the symptoms. If the patient is allergic to moulds, the reaction will be even more severe and last longer.

In addition, treatment to desensitise or neutralise any allergy to moulds and fungi or candida may actually cause a reaction instead of alleviating the symptoms. It is, therefore, important to know whether someone is allergic or not. Often we then choose to separate any desensitising or neutralising drops so the moulds are kept out of them. Then, after the antifungals have done their job, the vaccine for moulds is either added to the existing one, or a new one is made up and administered. Another way to avoid this problem is to use homeopathic preparations for the allergies and the candida.

Of course, the knowledge of an existing allergy or intolerance to candida and moulds is also helpful in monitoring the usefulness or otherwise of treatment. Sometimes people are treated with just a diet and supplements. This may or may not be enough. If it is not, then when we start the mould desensitising procedures, the patient will react which is a clear sign that the infection has not yet been successfully treated.

We then have the choice of persevering with the original treatment for a longer period; changing the remedy being used—often to a homeopathic one; or using an antifungal such as nystatin.

(Cont.)

A Case of Candida Allergy (Cont.)

Because an allergy to candida often spreads to include sensitivities to many environmental moulds and fungi, I organised to have several mould plates placed in Melissa's home and bedroom and asked the mycologists to analyse them. The report told me her bedroom was full of cladosporium, aspergillus, penicillium and had a light content of several other moulds and fungi.

At this point, we started to check her allergies. An immunoglobin E blood test turned out to be normal but a skin scratch test showed Melissa to be very sensitive to several moulds and fungi, especially TOE (trichophyton-mix, candida, pidermophytoninguinaie) aspergillus, penicillium, cladosporium and candida albicans.

I then explained to Melissa that she would have to be desensitised and would need to be particularly careful of mould exposure in both her environment and food. She followed my advice and within a few weeks Melissa was free of her symptoms.

Obviously not everyone with mood swings, irritability, anxiety, fatigue, skin and weight problems will have candida, hypoglycaemia, excessive histamine or a deficiency of ionised calcium, but these conditions are sufficiently prevalent to warrant a full analysis before toximolecular medicine is allowed to step in with powerful psychiatric drugs, addictive tranquillisers and other toxic medications.

3

MOOD SWINGS, TRANQUILLISERS AND NATURAL ALTERNATIVES

Millions of people, the majority of them women, take tranquillisers and other mood-altering drugs without quite knowing what they are or why they are taking them. Few people realise that in many, if not all, cases these medications, known as tranquillisers, are habit forming, cause side effects and don't work at all after a few months. For all practical purposes they are simply legal and socially acceptable drugs of addiction.

I have been practising nutritional medicine and psychiatry for more than a quarter of a century and during that time I have treated thousands of patients who have suffered with 'mental' or 'emotional' illnesses. I have rarely, if ever, seen anyone who has been cured by taking tranquillisers.

I have, however, seen patient after patient whose life has been ruined by becoming addicted to these drugs. I have also seen hundreds of people who, once they decide to stop taking tranquillisers, suffer withdrawal symptoms far worse than those which caused them to seek help in the first place.

In my clinical practice I have been able to help, advise and even cure many people whose allegedly 'mental' problems were, in fact, rooted in biochemical imbalances such as allergies, or physical illness, which responded admirably to dietary manipulations, nutrient supplementations, allergy treatment, anti-candida regimens or precursor (amino acids) therapy.

What are tranquillisers and how do they work?

There are literally hundreds of pharmaceutical and natural tranquillisers taken by millions of people all over the world in an attempt to relieve what is generally known as 'nervous tension'.

Tranquillisers are divided into two categories: minor and major tranquillisers. Minor tranquillisers are usually used for the relief of simple anxiety, muscle tension, sleeplessness and sometimes to buffer the withdrawal from illicit drugs or alcohol. The major ones are reserved for those who, in the opinion of the prescriber, suffer from a 'psychiatric' problem. Examples of the latter are schizophrenics, manic depressive psychotics and those with bipolar depression (also known as manic depression).

In addition, some of these drugs are short acting, which means that they produce an effect rather quickly but the effect is short-lived. In other words, you are unlikely to feel the effects of these medications one or two days after taking them. Other tranquillisers are medium acting and some are long acting.

Anyone wishing to give up taking tranquillisers should be aware that some of the drugs in all of the above groups have a short life in the body while others have a much longer life. Once again, this seemingly baffling differentiation has a simple meaning. In order to give up something one must decide whether to cut down gradually, or stop suddenly. Drugs that linger in the body for a long time (the long-life ones) need a very different timetable from the short-life ones, for obvious reasons, if one is to avoid, or at least minimise, the withdrawal effects.

There is also a great deal of confusion as to what tranquillisers can and cannot be used for. Most people do not realise that some sleeping pills are, in fact, tranquillisers taken in larger doses at bedtime. They include names such as Mogadon® or Dalmane®.

So, in order to familiarise yourself with mood-altering drugs, please have a good look at the descriptions that follow:

ANALGESICS

Names Codeine
Medical uses Painkiller, cough suppressant
Short-term effects of average dose Masks pain by creating mental clouding, drowsiness and, in some cases, mild to extreme euphoria.

NARCOTICS

Names Heroin, morphine, opium, methadone
Medical uses Analgesics, methadone is used for heroin addiction
Short-term effects of average dose Masks pain by creating mental clouding, drowsiness and mild to extreme euphoria. In contrast, some users experience nausea, vomiting and an itching sensation. Methadone's effects last considerably longer (24–36 hours compared with 2–4).
Short-term effects of large dose Same as average dose but of greater intensity. Insensitivity to pain is enhanced. A dreaming state of relaxation with total awareness but giving the appearance of sleep. In some cases, there is a paradoxical effect of increased energy and mental clarity. Overdoses produce unconsciousness, slow and shallow breathing, cold and clammy skin and a weak but fast pulse rate. When mixed with other depressants these may cause death.
Long-term effects of chronic use or abuse Physical addiction, lethargy, weight loss, difficulties with erection and ejaculation and a loss of libido (sexual interest).
Withdrawal symptoms Restlessness, irritability, tremors, anorexia (loss of appetite), panic, chills, sweating, cramps, watery eyes, runny nose, nausea, vomiting and muscle spasms.

BARBITURATES

Common trade names Amytal®, Nembutal®, Phenobarbital®, Seconal®
Medical uses Sedation, relief from tension, anaesthetic

(Cont.)

Barbiturates (Cont.)

Short-term effects of average dose Relaxation, sleep. Used recreationally, these drugs are a little like alcohol but without the calories. They produce mild intoxication, loss of inhibition (users could become sexually aggressive), decreased alertness and decreased muscle co-ordination.

Short-term effects of large dose All the effects of lower dose will be accentuated with the addition of slurred speech, shallow and slow breathing, cold and clammy skin, weak and rapid heart beat, and hangover feelings. Unconsciousness can move beyond sleep to coma and eventually death.

Long-term effects of chronic use or abuse Sleepiness, confusion, irritability, severe withdrawal sickness with symptoms such as anxiety, insomnia, tremors, delirium, convulsions and occasionally death. Tolerance to sedative effect increases so one may need to take larger doses to obtain the same effect. Unfortunately, the tolerance to lethal dose does not increase so that one may increase dose to fatal levels. Gluthetimide—common brand name Doriden®—is similar to barbiturates but because it is longer acting the effects of an overdose are more difficult to reverse. They can be fatal.

Many people who take tranquillisers do not really understand what they are, what they can and cannot do and what their long-term effects are. Even fewer people know how to give them up once they have taken them and whether or not there are any natural, safe alternatives.

The effects of medications collectively banded under the umbrella term 'tranquillisers' are not to create tranquillity by 'calming' a troubled mind.

Tranquillisers tend to suppress the whole personality of the long-term user and, at best, act only as a filter through which daily events are perceived as less threatening. It is to be clearly understood that *any* event which is perceived as stressful, such as disappointments, arguments or any kind of conflict, will undergo this 'filtering' action irrespective of whether the individual would normally be able to cope with it.

MINOR TRANQUILLISERS

Long acting International names—these are the international names or the names for the actual active chemical ingredients. They are not brand names. The same chemical can have different brand names in different countries and there can be several variants of the same chemicals. For example, benzodiazepine is a general group of tranquillisers, of which diazepam is one. The usual brand name for this is Valium®.

Bromazepam, chlordiazepoxide, colbazam, chlorazepate dipotassium, diazepam, flunitrazepam, flurazepam, nitrazepam. Some common brand names are: Librium®, Tranxene®, Valium®.

Medical uses Relief from anxiety, muscular tension and the symptoms of alcohol withdrawal.

Short-term effects of average dose Mild sedation, a sense of well-being and an increased ability to cope. May cause headaches and in rare cases can have a paradoxical effect of increasing anxiety and hostile behaviour.

Short-term effects of large dose Drowsiness, blurred vision, slurred speech, stupor. If mixed with alcohol, can cause suppression of breathing and even death.

Long-term effects of chronic use or abuse Impairment of sexual functions, confusion, irritability, severe withdrawal sickness which can appear several days after intake has stopped. Tolerance to sedative effect increases, so one may need to take larger doses to obtain the same effect.

Withdrawal symptoms Anxiety, insomnia, tremors, delirium, convulsions and occasionally death.

Medium acting Aprazolam, lorazepam, oxazepam, lormentazepam, temazepam. They have the same advantages and disadvantages of the long-acting tranquillisers.

In this way, the person taking the tranquillisers does not have the possibility of adjusting to the situation and is, therefore, denied any opportunity of learning to cope with what may well be a perfectly normal, everyday event.

Most people are prescribed tranquillisers because they have stresses in their lives with which they are not coping. These stresses may be emotional ones, such as problems at home or at work, or problems with money, or phobias and insecurities, or any number of factors that impact on our lives. There are also physical, bio-chemical and nutritional stresses which include allergies, chemical sensitivities, severe premenstrual tension, candida infections and post-viral syndrome.

Because life is so stressful, and people are often unwell without knowing exactly why, many tend to abuse tranquillisers to the point where they become addicted to them.

Addiction versus withdrawal

2001 poll carried out by the BBC's *Panorama* programme revealed that over one and a half million adults in the UK had been pre-scribed tranquilliser drugs long-term, in spite of government advice to GPs in 1988 that they should not prescribe more than a four-week supply of benzodiazepines. The investigation revealed that doctors are routinely prescribing drugs they know can cause addic-tion and which have a range of serious side effects. The poll results showed that 28 per cent of patients admitted to having been on the drugs for more than ten years.

Tranquillisers are supposed to calm you down; they are 'anxi-olytic' which is a medical term for anti-anxiety. Some doctors still believe that most people suffering from depression are also anxious and so often prescribe tranquillisers to these patients. In fact, there is no evidence that tranquillisers are of any use whatsoever against depression as such and many depressed people who take tranquillis-ers end up committing suicide.

So what symptoms are likely to prompt someone being pre-scribed tranquillisers? Here is a list of the most common ones: excessive sweating, panic attacks, palpitations, inability to sleep, shakiness, pins and needles, fearfulness, perceptual distortions, lack of concentration, lack of confidence and phobias.

As I said earlier, and as all medical textbooks tell us, tranquillisers should only be used for a short time. However, often people take them for months, even years on end and, when they try to stop, they find they cannot because they suffer withdrawal symptoms. They have become addicted.

What are the withdrawal symptoms that keep people taking their tranquillisers? Here is a short list of withdrawal symptoms: excessive sweating, panic attacks, palpitations, inability to sleep, shakiness, pins and needles, fearfulness, perceptual distortions, lack of concentration, lack of confidence, nightmares, hallucinations, convulsions.

No, this is not a misprint. The symptoms that cause someone to be prescribed tranquillisers are very similar to those that he or she will experience when trying to stop taking them!

People who have been taking tranquillisers for a while may decide to stop taking them. However, when they start to feel sick, to shake visibly, to experience anxiety attacks or to become so fearful that they cannot leave home, they go back to their doctor and are often prescribed larger doses of the tranquillisers that are causing their withdrawal symptoms. The next inevitable step is that the patient becomes totally dependent on the drugs and remains on them full time.

Because the symptoms experienced by patients when they try to stop taking tranquillisers can be quite severe, many people give up and continue taking them. However, the incidence and severity of withdrawal symptoms can be greatly reduced by following a well-planned programme that uses natural alternatives and other supportive therapy.

THE TRANQUILLISER CYCLE

If you are taking, or are thinking about taking tranquillisers, you should be aware of a few facts:

- Doctors often prescribe drugs, such as Valium®, Serepax®, Ducene®, Mogadon®, Euhypnos® or Rhohypnol®, to people who are worried, sad, panicky, or unable to sleep.
- These states are often caused by things such as divorce, grief, domestic violence, a boring job or one that is too demanding, money problems or many other physical stresses on your body.

(Cont.)

The Tranquilliser Cycle (Cont.)

- On some occasions taking tranquillisers may help you to get through a crisis situation; however, taking them regularly will not resolve your marriage, pay your rent or calm down an aggressive partner.
- All tranquillisers do is block out your feelings. Without feelings like anger, anxiety or sadness you are less likely to try to do something about resolving your problems and overcoming the crisis.
- Tranquillisers make your problems appear a little further away but they can also make you feel listless, affect your co-ordination and interfere with your ability to think clearly and therefore solve any problems!
- The longer you take tranquillisers, the less effect they have and so the only way you are able to keep calm or sleep easily is by taking more. Your body builds up a tolerance to the drug.
- Eventually you find that you cannot function very well without them and you are suffering from a dependency. You have become an addict.

Natural tranquillisers

As we have seen in the earlier part of this chapter, there are many reasons why tranquillisers are prescribed. Before any medication is prescribed, whether it is natural or otherwise, it is essential to find out the cause of the problem and whether, in fact, tranquillisers will benefit your condition.

There are a number of natural nutrients known as health supplements, which can help people and which can be taken instead of pharmaceutical tranquillisers. In many cases these natural alternatives are effective and they have few, if any, side effects. Like all medications, they need to be prescribed by a competent therapist who is thoroughly familiar with any possible problems that may be encountered.

Nowadays, there is an amazing array of supplements, such as vitamins, minerals and amino acids, available in health-food shops. Each one has a different claim: to cure this or that, to make you slim forever, or to keep you free from heart disease.

It is no wonder that many people are confused and disillusioned about what to expect from some of these natural alternatives. There is an increasing number of people who take supplements hoping that they will provide a 'miracle' cure for their ailments. Mental and physical health can at best be helped by supplements, it cannot be found in them!

Often, due to unsatisfactory results from these supplements, people consult with nutritional therapists to check that they are taking the right supplement, the right dose and that the primary cause of the problem has not been masked by their symptoms.

Following are some of the natural alternatives to tranquillisers. However, once again, it must be stressed that any supplements for any type of mood disorder should only be taken under professional supervision.

A former company director who says his life was ruined after he became addicted to Valium® has become one of the first people in the country to win damages after claiming he was negligently over-prescribed the drug. The powerful tranquilliser left him with severe side-effects including suicidal depression and panic attacks, forcing him to give up work in a nightmare which lasted more than a decade. He was put on a three-month programme to wean him off Valium® and has now won £40,000 in damages from his former GP.

Mike Waites, Health Correspondent,
Yorkshire Post, 27 June 2002

Phenylethylalanine

One of the body's natural antidepressants is phenylethylalanine. This is a chemical substance derived from phenylalanine which is a common amino acid found in many foods.

Phenylalanine is also used by the brain to make norepinephrine (noradrenaline) and to slow down the breakdown of the natural opiates (endorphins and enkephalines) which are responsible for, among other things, lowering the sensation of pain. Phenylalanine is sold as a supplement in the form of DL-phenylalanine (DLPA).

DL-phenylalanine (DLPA) may well revolutionise the treatment of depression and intractable pain. It can be a very successful method for the nutritional control of chronic depression and some types of pain.

Health professionals, pain treatment clinics and scientific research papers have reported dramatic results in patients with chronic depression, acute premenstrual syndrome symptoms and severe, acute and chronic-pain conditions, including rheumatoid arthritis, back pain, migraines and headaches, post-operative pain and neuralgia.

Phenylalanine is an 'essential' amino acid which exists in foods in two forms called D and L. It is most common in high-protein foods and we can metabolise and utilise it and its by-products quite easily. It is non-toxic and has been found to be ten times *less* toxic than Vitamin C.

DLPA analgesia requires anything from two to fourteen or more days to develop but its effects are long lasting. After initial treatment, the patient may need to take DLPA only a few days (typically about seven) every month. It works in what is probably the 'ideal' way, by intensifying and prolonging the body's natural painkillers (enkephalines and endorphins).

About twenty years ago it was discovered that the human brain synthesises a group of hormones with properties quite similar to morphine and opium. Appropriately, these were first called 'the brain's own opiates' and were found to follow the activation of pain signals. These endorphin hormones are part of a natural, built-in pain-relief system which is activated in cases of extreme stress. It is the system responsible for the loss of pain sensation when people who have suffered traumatic injuries find that they remain unaware of the extent of their problems for several hours after the event.

One of the problems with painkilling hormones, and indeed with many natural chemicals, is that there is an array of enzymes in the body ready to destroy them. DL-phenylalanine inhibits several enzymes which destroy these natural painkilling hormones. The inhibition of these enzymes enables painkillers to affect their influence for a much longer period of time.

Another important consideration is that people suffering chronic pain and depression tend to have lowered levels of endorphins. DLPA is thought to restore endorphin levels to normal and this would therefore allow the normal painkilling effects of the brain chemicals to continue for longer periods.

One of the great advantages of using natural substances as painkillers, rather than drugs, is that the normal, short-term signals

Foods containing phenylalanine

almonds	egg
apple	fish (herring)
avocado	milk
baked beans	parsley
banana	peanuts
beef	pineapple
beet	soya bean
carrot	soy proteins
chicken	spinach
cottage cheese	tomato
chocolate	

of acute pain, such as the result of hitting your thumb with a hammer or touching boiling water, are not inhibited.

Contraindications and warnings

While the use of a natural painkiller, such as phenylalanine, is still far safer than using pharmaceutical drugs, we must exercise extreme care when we start to tinker with the brain's chemistry.

At the Complementary and Environmental Medicine Centre we have conducted a series of trials and it appears that most of the claims for DLPA are indeed quite valid. We are, however, investigating its effects on behaviour and the preliminary conclusion is that it should be used with caution by people suffering from psychiatric disorders.

Dr Richard Wurtman, a neuroendocrinologist at the MIT, suggests that a rise in phenylalanine may completely block the normal rise in brain serotonin levels which follow the ingestion of certain meals. Wurtman's study shows that where serotonin levels are prevented from rising, this fools the brain into wanting more carbohydrates. One can only speculate at this point on the possible disruption in sleep patterns and mood changes which may occur because of this.

DLPA, and indeed *any* preparation containing phenylalanine, should not be taken by people suffering from phenylketonuria. It should not be taken during pregnancy and people suffering from hypertension (high blood pressure) are advised to take it *after* meals, instead of before meals (as it should normally be taken).

Magnesium

Too much nitrogen (fertilisers), excessive phosphorus (soft drinks) and too much copper (water pipes) and iron can cause an imbalance or deficiency of magnesium.

Dr Jerry Aikawa, of the University of Colorado Medical Centre, carried out several trials and achieved good results using magnesium as a tranquilliser.

When magnesium levels are too low, the nervous system becomes easily irritated. At some stage, an individual will experience feelings of disorientation and may even have convulsions. Muscular twitching is a common symptom and can be reversed by the administration of magnesium.

Magnesium can be such a powerful peripheral nervous system depressant that excessive doses can cause flaccid muscles and even a degree of anaesthesia. Patients with chronic insomnia, nervous tension, anxiety and muscular tension have been repeatedly found to have low levels of magnesium in their blood.

The calming effects of this mineral have also been proven in animals, thus counteracting claims of placebo influence. Dr Aikawa treated a group of thoroughbred horses, forty-one in all, of which two were known to be quite edgy. An analysis of the horses' blood showed that almost all the nervous ones had low magnesium levels in their blood. Once this mineral was added to their diet, the animals calmed down considerably.

Foods high in magnesium

almonds	barley
apricots, dried	beef
avocado	Brazil nuts
baked beans	carrots (raw)

(Cont.)

Food high in magnesium (Cont.)

cashews	peanuts
chicken	peas
citrus fruits	pecans
corn	pork
crab	potato
dates	rice
fish (flounder,	sesame
salmon, tuna)	soya beans
lentils	tomato (raw)
Lima beans	vegetables (dark green,
molasses	leafy ones)
oatmeal	wheat germ
peaches	

Vitamin B₁ (thiamine)

An article from the medical journal *Modern Medicine in Australia* described how a group of patients with symptoms such as sleeplessness, personality changes, aggressiveness and irritability were found to be deficient in Vitamin B_1. All the patients appeared to suffer with anxiety and every one of them responded to Vitamin B_1 supplements with either a complete remission of symptoms or a marked improvement in their moods. Vitamin B_1 acts as a coenzyme in the breakdown of carbohydrates by oxidising pyruvic acid. If there is not sufficient Vitamin B_1 available, pyruvic acid accumulates. This then becomes lactic acid which is eventually turned into lactate.

The connection between lactate and anxiety is well documented. We know that high blood levels or an unusual sensitivity to this natural by-product of muscular exertion and sugars can cause anxiety attacks in susceptible people. A hereditary predisposition or early liver damage may cause some people to experience a continuous low-level background anxiety state.

This condition is known as lactate induced anxiety syndrome (LIAS) (see page 43) and can often be treated successfully with large amounts of supplementary calcium, Vitamin B_1 and dietary manipulations to reduce pyruvic acid.

As well as being in excessive demand during periods of high carbohydrate consumption, Vitamin B_1 is destroyed by food processing methods such as heating and oxidation.

Foods high in Vitamin B_1 (thiamine)

beef (heart, liver, kidney)
Brazil nuts
cereals
fish (mackerel, perch,
   red snapper)
lamb
milk
oatmeal
peas and other legumes

pork (liver)
poultry
pumpkin
soya bean
sunflower seeds
wheat
wheat germ
yeast (Brewer's)

Alkalis also destroy Vitamin B_1. People taking stomach alkalisers (antacids) often find that they become irritable which increases stomach acidity, ulcer pains and abdominal discomfort. They then need more antacids or alkalisers, and a vicious circle is thus established. The next step is mental confusion and depression.

Studies have shown that Vitamin B_1 deficiencies in children may result in lowered IQ levels. (*Nutrition*, H. Guthrie, Professor of Nutrition, Pennsylvania State University, C.V. Mosby, pp. 259–320).

A growing number of young people—especially women—are addicted to over-the-counter medicines which help them cope with the stresses of everyday life. More than 30,000 people in Britain are said to be hooked on drugs that contain opiates and stimulants which can be bought at high street chemists without a prescription.

Independent on Sunday, 3 January 1999

Vitamin B_{12} (cyanocobalamine)

A deficiency of this vitamin is known to cause pernicious anaemia. What some people do not realise is that Vitamin B_{12} deficiencies are also associated with depression, neurosis, some forms of schizophrenia and psychosis.

Low Vitamin B_{12} levels, or histapenia, also cause a rise in pyruvic acid and, as we have seen, this can lead to increased circulating lactate and a state of anxiety. The similarity with Vitamin B_1, however, ends there.

Any of the following factors can contribute to a Vitamin B_{12} deficiency: malabsorption, irritable bowel syndrome, low stomach acidity, excessive intake of antacids, insufficient intrinsic factor, prolonged strict vegetarian diet (vegan), alcohol abuse and/or several prescribed medications such as anti-convulsants.

People suffering from emotional disorders associated with Vitamin B_{12} deficiency are known as histapenics because of the low levels of brain histamine (another neurotransmitter) which such a condition can cause. (For more information on histapenics see page 40.)

Foods high in Vitamin B_{12} (cyanocobalamine)

beef (kidney, liver)	pork (heart, liver)
cheese (cheddar, cream)	prunes
chicken	salmon
egg yolk	sardines
herring	shellfish
mackerel	tuna
milk	yoghurt

Vitamin B_6 (pyridoxine)

Gamma aminobutyric acid (GABA) is one of the neurotransmitters responsible for slowing down the chemical activity in the brain. Another neurotransmitter, glutamic acid is responsible for exciting chemical activity.

The manufacture of GABA is particularly reliant on ample supplies of Vitamin B_6 and for this reason alone Vitamin B_6 is often useful as a tranquilliser.

However, there is another important factor which also helps to explain the role of Vitamin B_6 and its sedating effects. GABA (the inhibitory neurotransmitter) is made from glutamic acid (the excitatory neurotransmitter) in the presence of Vitamin B_6. So, if there is too little Vitamin B_6, less GABA is made and the levels of glutamic acid rise thus causing irritability of the central nervous system. However, if there is ample Vitamin B_6, then a lot of GABA is made which helps in sedating or 'calming down' the brain.

At the same time, an excess of Vitamin B_6 could deplete glutamic acid reserves to the point where proper excitation and hence perception functions of the nervous system may be impaired.

For more information on GABA, glutamic acid and Vitamin B_6, see page 24.

Foods high in Vitamin B_6 (pyridoxine)

avocado	milk
barley	molasses
beans	oranges
Brazil nuts	peanuts
carrot	peas
cheese	potato
cow's milk	prunes
crab	rice
egg	soya bean
fish (cod, halibut, herring, mackerel, salmon, sardines, tuna)	spinach
	sunflower seeds
lentils	wheat bran
Lima beans	wheat germ
liver (pork)	wholemeal flour
meat (beef, ham, pork)	yeast (Brewer's)

Zinc

This mineral has a calming effect on our nerves and it also counteracts copper. Because of the widespread use of copper water pipes, many orthomolecular scientists feel that some individuals may suffer an overload of this mineral.

Foods high in zinc

beef (liver)	mushrooms
bran	oatmeal
Brazil nuts	oysters
crab	pork
egg	pumpkin seeds
grains	rice, brown
herring	sunflower seeds
kidney	tuna
lamb	veal
milk	yeast (Brewer's)

Copper happens to excite the nervous system and this may be one of the reasons why zinc is a very useful adjunct to the use of other natural tranquillisers.

Frozen vegetables are usually deficient in zinc. Some diets high in soya phytates may cause poor absorption of zinc. Alcohol abuse often creates a zinc deficiency as does anything that tends to irritate the gut lining, including antibiotics, food allergies and candida infestations.

Vitamic C (ascorbic acid)

Most people associate Vitamin C with the treatment or prevention of the common cold, influenza and viral infections.

What is far less well known is the fact that although brain cells cannot make Vitamin C, the concentration of this vitamin in the brain is higher than in any organ except the adrenal glands (the glands responsible for our responses to stress).

According to the pioneer of orthomolecular psychiatry himself, Dr Abraham Hoffer, Vitamin C is as active as some of the most powerful psychiatric medications in use today simply because it acts as a dopamine receptor blocker.

Weight for weight, it does the job as effectively as Haldol®, a dopamine antagonist widely used in the treatment of various forms of psychosis. High levels of dopamine in the brain are associated with aggressiveness, irritability and a host of psychiatric conditions such as schizophrenia.

Foods high in Vitamin C (ascorbic acid)

alfalfa	guava
banana	kidney
berries (blueberries, gooseberries,	liver (beef)
raspberries and strawberries)	oysters
Brazil nuts	potato
broccoli	spinach
Brussels sprouts	sweet potato
cantaloupe melon	vegetables
capsicum	(green leafy ones)
cauliflower	watermelon
citrus fruit (lemons, oranges, tomatoes)	

In order that Vitamin C may be effective in the brain, it has to be administered in huge doses so that at least a little will be forced, by mass action, to cross the blood-brain barrier.

> Thirty-four per cent of British women have been prescribed tranquillisers or sleeping pills at some time . . . Seventy-five per cent of the thirteen million prescriptions written annually for tranquillisers are for women. This means that every year nearly ten million women take tranquillisers.
>
> Dr Norma Williams and Hetty Einzig,
> *The New Guide to Women's Health*, 1985

Vitamin B₃

Vitamin B_3

There are two types of Vitamin B_3 and each one has two names: niacin, also known as nicotinic acid, and niacinamide, also known as nicotinamide.

In 1979, H. Mohler and his research group at Hoffman-La-Roche (the Swiss pharmaceutical company responsible for Valium®) discovered that nicotinamide is: ' . . . a brain constituent with benzodiazepine-like activity. . . . only nicotinamide showed the main neuropharmacological central effects characteristic of benzodiazepines although, because only 0.3 per cent enters the brain, rather high doses are needed to elicit effects.'

Benzodiazepine is the technical name for a group of chemicals that are used as minor tranquillisers such as Valium®. In order for Vitamin B_3 to be effective in any central nervous system activity, it has to be administered in megadoses so that at least a little will be forced, by mass action, to cross the blood-brain barrier.

Because nicotinamide has properties in common with Valium® and barbiturates this clearly indicates that it may be valuable as an anticonvulsant muscle relaxant, especially when administered together with magnesium, and as a general tranquilliser.

These are some of the reasons why we sometimes prescribe megadoses of Vitamin B_3. We know only too well that such high doses are needed to achieve any effect within the central nervous system.

Nicotinic acid (niacin) has quite different properties: it is very helpful as part of any treatment programme for most schizophrenias, senility and alcoholism but does not appear to have the same tranquillising effects of niacinamide. This is probably because the naturally occurring form of Vitamin B_3 in the human body is nicotinamide dinucleotide (NAD) which contains niacinamide, not niacin.

Inositol

A little known nutrient factor usually assumed to be a part of the B-group vitamins has been reported by some therapists to exert a powerful tranquillising effect.

4

DEPRESSION

Gloom and doom, sadness and madness, melancholy, the doldrums, languor, sorrowfulness—depression has many names and is often described as the common cold of psychiatry. It is a very common problem and, indeed, it is a rare individual who does not feel depressed at some time or another.

When psychiatrists speak of depression, however, they are talking about a clinical state of illness of which there are many types, and each kind of depression can have several symptoms.

The type of depression diagnosed will depend on the symptoms, an analysis of the patient's history and perhaps some psychological or other tests. Then, a suitable treatment is prescribed. Unfortunately, even though it sounds quite simple, it is not.

Depression can be unipolar or 'simple', or bipolar. Bipolar depression is also known as manic depression and a variation of it is called manic depressive psychosis (MDP). There is also a variation of MDP known as seasonal affective disorder syndrome (SADS). There is also post partum depression (PPD) as well as endogenous (from within or spontaneous, if you prefer) and reactive depression.

Reactive depression means you are depressed because *that* is the way you react to something that has happened to you. Although endless lists of such causes of reactive depression are regularly compiled by psychologists, the fact is that some things affect some people more than others. Some of us seem to shrug off adverse events while others become depressed every time things don't run smoothly. Given the infinite variety of humans, this is entirely understandable. It is only when an individual fails to recover after the causative event has passed, that such a permanently depressed state becomes a clinical illness.

Most of us find the many labels and terms used by psychologists and psychiatrists very confusing and not particularly helpful in finding the root of the depression.

Depression can be caused by almost anything: lowered immune responses, candida, alcohol abuse or over-indulgence, Vitamin B_{12} deficiency, an imbalance or deficiency of several minerals, nutrients and amino acids, different kinds of anaemia, malabsorption, hypoglycaemia or food allergies.

Depressed people can become obsessive or indolent, lackadaisical or compulsive, lazy or workaholics. In fact, the range of individual reactions to depression is almost as varied as human nature. The only thing they all have in common is the depression. There are, of course, some well known causes for depression.

It is often the case that many people who suffer from depression are also overweight. The therapist must always try to assess if any particular individual is depressed *because* he or she is overweight or whether it is the other way around. The fact is that the two seem to go hand in hand.

Special assessment tests, such as the Hoffer and Osmond diagnostic test, are well suited to detecting true clinical depression. Following are some of the reasons why depression can lead to weight gain and a discussion about some of the common causes of depression.

Touching, tyrosine, depression and weight gain

Nowadays we know that stress in general can cause the body's levels of noradrenaline (also called norepinephrine) to become exhausted. Low levels of noradrenaline are associated with depression. Using drugs that do not elevate noradrenaline levels for this type of depression will not help alleviate the problem.

Therapists familiar with nutritional (orthomolecular) psychiatry also know that otherwise useful nutrients, such as Vitamin B_6, tryptophan and zinc, and high complex carbohydrate diets, such as vegetarianism or Pritikin, will not usually resolve this type of depression and may, in some cases, make it worse. Conversely, we know that whenever stress is a strong contributing factor in clinical depression, tyrosine is probably the treatment of choice.

Depression often, but not always, goes hand in hand with low blood pressure, low blood sugar, low thyroid functions (all of which tend to contribute to weight gain), and low adrenal gland functions.

Foods containing tyrosine

alfalfa	cucumber
almonds	egg
apple	fig
apricot	fish (herring)
asparagus	leek
avocado	lettuce
baked beans	milk
banana	parsley
beef	peanuts
beet	poultry
capsicum	soya bean
carrot	soy proteins
cheese	spinach
cherries	strawberries
chicken	watercress
chocolate	watermelon
cottage cheese	yoghurt

Tyrosine can normalise blood pressure, stimulate the thyroid and contribute to blood-sugar stabilisation via adrenal support. Patients suffering with this kind of depression often crave many different types of foods and while these may include sweets, there can also be a strong desire for cheese, chocolate and other tyrosine-containing foods.

If digestion is impaired (as in low hydrochloric acid states or intestinal candidiasis, for example), then dietary tyrosine is converted to tyramine. Tyramine stimulates the adrenal glands and causes further depletion of noradrenaline stores, while at the same time depriving glands like the thyroid of needed tyrosine. The following diagram shows us this relationship.

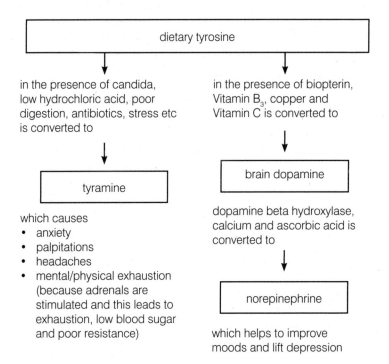

Tyrosine is one of the three aromatic amino acids (the other two are phenylalanine and tryptophan) which cross the blood-brain barrier. Levels of tyrosine in the brain are somewhat dependent on dietary intake. However, just taking tyrosine supplements is not enough to increase levels.

Like most amino acids, tyrosine transport from the blood to the brain is highly competitive with other amino acids—especially the branched amino acids (leucine, isoleucine and valine). Along with tryptophan, all these amino acids inhibit the brain's uptake of tyrosine. So tyrosine is more likely to be beneficial if taken on an empty stomach.

The metabolism of tyrosine is dependent on a form of folic acid (biopterin) and a type of Vitamin B_3 (NADH) as well as copper and Vitamin C. Once tyrosine reaches the neurons, it is converted to dopamine and then norepinephrine which helps lift depression.

This last, but crucial, step, however, depends on the presence of an enzyme (tyrosine hydroxylase) at the pre-synaptic nerve ending. The availability of the enzyme, and therefore the output of useful norepinephrine, depends on the amount of electrical activity along the nerve.

Now, if *anything* touches you, nerve impulses are transmitted from the point of impact to the brain. Therefore, chiropractic, osteopathy, massage, acupuncture, caressing, touching or any physical contact will cause an increase of electrical nerve impulses. This will increase the amount of the enzyme, tyrosine hydroxylase, which is necessary to produce the anti-depressant neurotransmitter chemical—norepinephrine.

In addition, tyrosine is the precursor of the thyroid hormone. Low thyroid function tends to go hand in hand with high oestrogen and not enough Vitamin E. This combination makes for poor circulation, weight gain, a slow metabolism and lack of libido.

There is very little tyrosine in cereals, grains, fruit, vegetables or oils. The highest concentrations are to be found in wild game and yoghurt.

THE CASE OF MARY X

This patient was referred to me because she was suffering with depression, digestive disturbances, such as bloating and intestinal gas, as well as diarrhoea and constipation. She was grossly overweight but denied overeating and was not particularly fond of sweets. She tended to be anxious, fearful and somewhat shaky. Her mental state was one of confusion and she described herself as 'unable to cope'. Her skin tended to be dry, her menstrual blood was often clotty, she suffered with recurrent skin rashes, her breasts became sensitive before her period and she felt the cold easily and always complained of icy hands and feet.

(Cont.)

The Case of Mary X (Cont.)

She displayed many of the symptoms of hypothyroidism (low thyroid function). A basal temperature test confirmed this fact. The original diagnosis, made by the referring practitioner, had been of candida (systemic thrush) and indeed, a yeast-free diet coupled with antifungal medications did improve most of her digestive symptoms and her skin. However, she still had difficulties losing weight and was still very depressed and somewhat anxious.

Mary was under a great deal of personal stress in her relationship and her mother had recently passed away. A blood test confirmed that she had a mild yeast infection but when I analysed the results I also discovered her immune system was working reasonably well and taking care of that situation.

I asked Mary to attend a competent masseur and suggested that she have a massage every day. I also told her to ask her partner to give her plenty of cuddles. Keeping the whole thing in a somewhat light vein, I discussed the matter with her partner and explained that Mary was not 'neurotic' or in any way mentally ill but that she suffered from a number of biochemical and nutritional problems which could easily be overcome. I assured him she would soon be well and explained that his co-operation would make this happen much faster.

In addition to extra hugging and touching, Mary was prescribed supplements of tyrosine to be taken in the morning and again mid-morning—always on an empty stomach. Within four weeks Mary had lost 3 kilograms, she was no longer depressed and most of her anxiety was a thing of the past.

Tyrosine tends to elevate blood pressure in people suffering with low blood pressure and lower it in those suffering with high blood pressure: it exerts an adaptogenic and normalising effect.

Contraindications and warnings

Tyrosine, as with most aromatic amino acids, may be contraindicated in some types of schizophrenia. Orthomolecular practitioners are well aware of the contraindications of amino acid supplementation in psychosis and assess each patient very carefully before administering megadoses.

Psychiatric assessment tests, such as the Hoffer and Osmond diagnostic test, coupled with a thorough medical history and as many details as possible about the effects of previous medications, are all carefully considered. In some cases, of course, it is quite reasonable to carry out short trials with different amino acids because the response, or lack of it, usually indicates the underlying biochemical problem.

Treatment of this type should only be followed under the strict guidance of a qualified practitioner in orthomolecular nutrition who is familiar with this type of orthomolecular psychiatry (also known as precursors therapy).

On the other hand, most of the beneficial effects of tyrosine, or the side effects of an overdose, can be wiped out by the simultaneous administration of large amounts of neutral amino acids. Caffeine tends to lower plasma levels of tyrosine and could therefore increase the effects of stress in general.

TYROSINE AND CANCER

The idea that certain types of cancer need specific amino acids to thrive is not a new one. As far back as the 1960s trials were carried out with low phenylalanine diets in an attempt to 'starve' cancer cells. Success with this treatment was less than hoped for.

There are certain forms of cancer, such as malignant melanomas and glioblastoma multiforma, where the cancer cells are known to soak up tyrosine at a great rate. It would be prudent, therefore, not to use this amino acid under those circumstances unless the possible advantages clearly outweigh the potential risk.

Tryptophan and depression

Of course, there are some types of depression which respond poorly, or not at all, to tyrosine and need tryptophan instead.

The clues to non-tyrosine-dependent depressions are quite simple: sufferers will invariably crave sweets and consume carbohydrates (complex or otherwise) at every opportunity. Whenever they feel hungry, and this is usually mid-afternoon and late evenings, they will choose carbohydrates. They will often have gigantic sandwiches at ungodly hours. It is not the filling that is important, only the bread!

As a general rule, these depressed patients tend to have sleeping problems and usually respond well to tryptophan, another amino acid which crosses into the brain via the blood-brain barrier.

Tryptophan also comes from proteins but, unlike tyrosine, it requires the simultaneous presence of carbohydrates in order to enter the brain. Once it has entered the brain, tryptophan is then changed into serotonin which is a neurotransmitter that can lift some types of depression, induce drowsiness and stimulate immune functions.

Interestingly, the same combination of carbohydrates craving and depression can also be found in people suffering from bulimia and several types of premenstrual syndrome. Many cases of premenstrual syndrome respond well to oral supplements of tryptophan.

It is also interesting to note that many antidepressants cause people to gain weight and scientists spent some time searching for a drug that did not cause this side effect. Fluoxetine (brand name Prozac®) heralded a new class of antidepressant medications, and guess what? It exerts its antidepressant effect by artificially increasing brain levels of serotonin (the product of tryptophan).

THE CASE OF PAMELA X

Pamela was suffering from premenstrual tension (PMT) and depression during her period. After interviewing her, I decided her premenstrual syndrome was not caused predominantly by tension but by a combination of high levels of oestrogen and depression. She was also overweight and craved sweets, especially before her periods.

Pamela found it difficult to fall asleep, yet she needed lots of sleep in order to function at work; something she found herself less and less capable of doing. Her libido was all but gone and her husband's flowers and dinners were doing nothing to encourage a sexual spark on Pamela's part.

(Cont.)

The Case of Pamela X (Cont.)

I prescribed a B-complex formula and plenty of primrose oil and tryptophan in tablet form to be taken at bedtime on an empty stomach, together with a teaspoon of honey. I also gave her magnesium to be taken daily starting half way through her menstrual cycle, and regular doses of Vitamin E and calcium.

Three months later Pamela's depression had ceased, she had lost weight and her libido had returned.

Foods containing tryptophan

alfalfa	egg
baked beans	endive
beef	fennel
beet	fish
broccoli	milk
Brussels sprouts	nuts
carrot	soya bean
cauliflower	spinach
celery	sweet potato
chicken	turkey
chive	turnip
cottage cheese	watercress

Sunlight and depression

The science that deals with our biological clocks and rhythms is called chronobiology. It is a growing area of research, and recent findings suggest that the actual timing of food intake, sleep patterns and even the hour at which drugs are administered may be a great deal more important than we have previously thought.

I am sure most of you know that we are supposed to experience a lift in moods in spring. It's the time of the year when our hormones are supposed to get up and get going and drive us towards such human follies as chasing members of the opposite sex and other hedonistic lapses of good sense.

This notion, buried deeply in folklore, has a lot of truth in it. As the days get longer and the hours of darkness start later, wild flowers poke their heads above the ground, the winter blues vanish and new bursts of energy seem available on demand. This often happens to people who spend almost all the winter months in a state of mental hibernation—a sort of mind-slush which slows them down and makes them feel depressed.

We now know that many people who suffer the blues all winter but obtain a reprieve every spring suffer from seasonal affective disorder syndrome (SADS). The cause of their problems, their yearly spontaneous recovery, is linked to their pineal gland.

THE PINEAL GLAND AND NATURE

Nearly all reptiles, amphibians, birds, fish and mammals have a pineal gland and the few that do not have cells that perform the same functions.

The pineal gland has been part of the animal world for at least 500 million years and organs as ancient and widespread as it are not there for the evolutionary ride alone.

The importance of the functions of this little gland can be gathered by observing that when it is surgically removed it alters the physiology and behaviour of any animal profoundly. Breeding cycles go haywire, or stop altogether. Fish lose their protective colourings, making them easy victims of predators. Frogs and squirrels are no longer able to adjust their body temperature and birds lose the desire to migrate. Even deer are affected by growing antlers at the wrong time.

The pineal gland seems to adjust the whole physiology of animals to their environment.

Named because of its shape—it is a little like a pine-cone—the pineal gland is smaller than an aspirin tablet and it is now recognised as the seat of our biological clock. It is the organ responsible for our daily rhythms (circadian), most animals' mating seasons and also the daily and seasonal changes in biochemical functions.

The pineal gland is a 'neuroendocrinal transducer'—it translates input signals, such as light, into nerve impulses which in turn stimulate endocrinal glands to produce a veritable cascade of hormones.

These hormones control, affect and modify almost all aspects of animal physiology, biochemistry and behaviour. When light signals are scarce or absent, the pineal gland activates two of its resident enzymes: N-acetyl transferase (NAT) and hydroxyindole-O-methyltransferase (HIOMT). These enzymes then begin to turn serotonin into the hormone melatonin. If you are susceptible, and SADS sufferers obviously are, the resulting lack of serotonin makes you depressed. With the coming of spring and more daylight, the process is reversed and there is a lift in mood.

As a result of the process shown above, more serotonin is available to curb appetite in general and carbohydtates and sweets in particular. One sleeps better and tends to be less depressed

In spite of all the important functions the pineal gland has, it is not, as once believed, the master at all. It is, in fact, a slave under the control of yet another 'master clock': the suprachiasmatic nuclei. This mass of specialised brain cells, thankfully described as SCN, controls the pineal gland's nightly output of NAT.

Many animals hibernate during winter and it is also the end of any mating urges animals have. It is now believed that the hibernation process is triggered by melatonin and, as we have seen, the brain uses serotonin to make melatonin.

As daylight hours become shorter, the pineal produces more melatonin and the incidence of SADS depression increases. Apart from being a good reason for extending daylight-saving, it is interesting to note that increased serotonin plays a role in stimulating the immune system.

Have you ever noticed that when you are ill, especially when you have a viral disease such as a bad case of the 'flu, you tend to sleep a lot. The body knows your immune system needs a little boosting and increases serotonin levels which makes you sleepy. This in turn makes you conserve your energy and so the cycle goes on.

Knowing that sunshine decreases melatonin and therefore increases serotonin levels in the brain may help to explain why excessive sunbaking can make you so sleepy, while a brisk walk on a clear day can make you feel more alert.

Sunlight versus artificial light

Artificial light, especially fluorescent lights, are not as good as natural light. To produce the required effects of natural light, full-spectrum lights should be used. Millions of people, especially in colder climates, spend a great part of their daily lives under some form of artificial light. Light bulbs emit light which differs greatly from sunshine. Sunlight casts a full range of colours as well as ultraviolet and infrared light. Incandescent light bulbs emit only the yellow, orange and red portions of the spectrum.

Fluorescent lights work by passing a current through a tube filled with argon gas and mercury vapour which gives off a bluish light. Fluorescent lights can be made to give off any combination of colours; however, early developers decided to use the yellow and green portions of the spectrum because the human eye is most sensitive to them. This gives the characteristic 'cool-white' light with which we are all familiar.

Photobiologists are now finding that spending a lot of time exposed to only 'cool-white' portions of the light spectrum can upset the delicate human biochemistry by altering the ratio of hormones. It can also cause calcium malabsorption and deficiencies as well as a need for additional Vitamin A. Unshielded fluorescent light may also add ultraviolet radiation and so sensitive people may become more susceptible to skin cancer.

THE CASE OF JOHN X

John was referred to me by one of my ex-students. 'John is clearly suffering from hypoglycaemia', my ex-student told me over the phone. 'If he goes for as little as four hours without a meal he suffers headaches, brain fag and becomes extremely moody. Yet when I asked him to avoid refined carbohydrates and increase protein intake, he became very tired and depressed. I changed his diet to include more complex carbohydrates and he improved somewhat but gained weight. He then had to go away on business for a few weeks (in the middle of winter) and by the time he got back he was suicidal!'

John explained to me that as soon as he arrived at his destination he became almost frantic about finding some ice cream. Unless he had some sweets, he would become terribly depressed. His job kept him indoors almost all day and, when he got to his hotel at night, he spent several hours working under artificial light.

John was suffering from SADS. I prescribed supplemental tryptophan, calcium, Vitamin A and Vitamin B_3 and suggested that he spend at least a couple of hours each day walking around in the open air. I also explained to him that he should not spend too much time under fluorescent lighting and should attempt to change his home and office lights to the full-spectrum variety.

Chemicals and depression

Ask anyone what they think are the causes of depression and you will hear many similar answers: lack of money, overwork, unhappy relationships, stress—the list goes on. Ask a professional with a general knowledge of science and medicine and the list will be similar, but with extra things such as hereditary factors, brain malfunctions or severe illness. Doctors or psychiatrists will add various complex brain-chemical (neurotransmitter) imbalances, childhood traumas and several diseases to that list.

If, however, you were to talk to an experienced environmental medicine practitioner or to an orthomolecular psychiatrist, you would learn that depression can also be caused by allergies, or intolerances, to a variety of foods, inhalants and chemicals, or nutritional imbalances or deficiencies of vitamins, minerals and amino acids. There is also a variety of seemingly unrelated conditions, such as candida infections, irritable bowel syndrome and post-viral syndrome, which can cause depression. Long-term, low-grade exposure to toxic, foreign chemicals (xenobiotics) whether you are allergic to them or not, can also cause depression. (Naturally, the same applies to short-term overexposure.)

Profound sensitivity syndrome

While we all meet people who are emotionally *very* sensitive (the type that cries at the drop of a hat), there appears to be a certain proportion of the population who are profoundly sensitive to a vast array of factors in their environment. This problem is called profound sensitivity syndrome (PSS). People suffering from PSS are usually creative, artistic, highly perceptive and emotionally sensitive.

Some believe that people with PSS are more likely to suffer from auto-immune diseases such as lupus, multiple sclerosis and arthritis. Because PSS sufferers perceive many events as stressful that others would consider trivial, they often suffer the physical consequences of chronic, low-grade stress. Environmental doctors have added a new dimension to this proposition. They argue, convincingly in my opinion and clinical experience, that people who are inherently emotionally hypersensitive are more likely to be susceptible to environmental pollutants and xenobiotics. Often, in fact, neuropsychiatric symptoms such as depression, anxiety and paranoia are the first noted manifestations of some physical illness.

Hereditary factors, past illness or lifestyle can make some people's nervous system more susceptible to viral or chemical agents. Usually, such damage manifests itself as mood swings, agitation, feeling 'spaced out', poor concentration and memory impairment. All these are signs of central nervous system depression.

Environmental illness specialists also believe that chemical sensitivity can be transmitted from mother to child. Dr William Rae, founder and director of the Environmental Health Centre in Dallas, Texas, says:

> You can pass down chemicals and sensitivities from mother to child. It's seen in dope addicts and their babies, cigarette smokers and their babies and alcoholics and their babies. So it's not really startling that other chemicals are passed down. It's the logical extension. The data is there. If the mother had ten parts of styrene (a highly toxic xenobiotic compound which some plastic coffee cups and some insulation materials are made of) in her blood, the child may have two, or three parts in his.

As a result of a parent's sensitivity, a child may be born with a predisposition towards profound sensitivity. Dr Rae explains that conventional doctors and psychiatrists do not understand the interactions between the environment and human beings. In his experience, a third of his depressed patients are so because they have been exposed to chloroform. He has tested thousands of depressed patients and, in many cases, found high levels of chloroform in their blood. Similar results have also been found in Australia.

Chloroform is an anaesthetic and is in the steamy vapours which arise from the chlorine in our water during a long, hot shower. Now you know why a hot shower can be so relaxing and sleep inducing, while a cold one tends to be invigorating.

What a lot of people don't know is that many solvents, such as trichloroethane (used in dry cleaning and many other industrial cleaning applications) can also affect your mental state and cause mood swings, depression and even anxiety.

Another little-known fact is that many of these chemicals are partially alcohols and that the body mechanisms for clearing them share the same pathways as alcohol, which is a central nervous system depressant. Because air pollution can contain staggering amounts (100 tons per year in the air of Dallas alone) of such xenobiotics and because our detox pathways (mainly via the liver) are already very busy taking care of alcohol and many other xenobiotics, it is hardly surprising that depression is common.

Another xenobiotic that can precipitate depression, as well as other symptoms, is formaldehyde. It can affect the nervous system of profoundly sensitive people causing depression, poor concentration, memory problems and agitation.

How can we get such chemicals into our blood? Consider the following. If you place a lemon on a table a metre away, chances are you will be able to smell its fragrance. The reason is that the lemon, like everything else, decomposes ever so slightly, so that minute particles are inhaled—hence you can smell it.

Anything that can be smelled eventually enters your bloodstream. This process is known as 'outgassing'. So, if your new carpet, plastic fabric or furniture outgasses, chances are some formaldehyde enters your blood. If you are profoundly sensitive, it can cause depression.

Depression and other emotional problems can also be caused by old viruses: viruses which one may have contracted years, even decades, before without them exhibiting symptoms at the time. When such viruses are re-activated, mood swings and emotional problems can occur. This is also caused by post-viral syndrome.

Fatigue, depression and adrenal exhaustion

Poor adrenal functions, excessively low cholesterol levels and a lack of salt are often overlooked as a possible cause for depression and tiredness.

When the adrenals do not work as well as they should, the condition is known as chronic adrenal insufficiency, the burnout syndrome, hypoadrenia or hypoadrenocorticism.

It is not uncommon to find symptoms such as low blood pressure, hypoglycaemia, impaired liver function and salt cravings in people who have impaired or insufficient adrenal functions.

The adrenal glands consist of two parts: an outer, tough exterior called the cortex, and an interior part called the medulla. The medulla produces the hormone called adrenaline. The adrenal medulla and the cortex are both under the control of the pituitary gland, which sits at the base of the brain and is itself controlled by the hypothalamus.

The hypothalamus is a tiny pocket, or ventricle, in the brain which acts like a bugging device on all incoming messages about sight, sound, taste and smell. It translates these messages into chemical substances called releasing factors, and the releasing factors cause the pituitary gland to give off appropriate hormones, some of which affect the adrenal glands.

Hypoglycaemia

When the body is under stress, the adrenal glands secrete glucocorticoids which result in an increase in blood-sugar levels. The pancreas has to secrete insulin to cope with the increased blood sugar and levels return to normal.

If, however, this happens too often, then both the adrenals and the pancreas are forced to work overtime. The pancreas may also over-react in these situations causing blood-sugar levels to be constantly low (hypoglycaemia). Low blood sugar is one possible cause for chronic fatigue.

It also stands to reason that if one's adrenals are working below par—as is often the case when one has been under stress for a long time—tiredness will be one of the inevitable results.

Salt

Another consequence of exhausted adrenals and many acute illnesses is that blood levels of sodium (salt) decrease.

The adrenals, which are in charge of this department too, pour out special hormones, called mineralocorticoids, to help the body retain whatever salt it gets from the diet. At the same time, there is an excessive loss of potassium. If we eat too much salt, the result can be fluid retention and other complications; if there is not enough salt in the food we eat, the adrenals have to work much harder and their efficiency suffers further.

Most doctors and many nutritionists consider that we already have too much salt in our diet. Yet many seem unaware that the connection between dietary salt and high blood pressure is not only far from proven but that there is much scientific evidence showing that only a small percentage of people, specifically those who are sensitive to sodium, will have their blood pressure increased by dietary salt intake.

Much attention is given to high blood pressure and risks of cardiovascular disease. However, very little publicity is given to the very common condition of low blood pressure.

Low blood pressure can make people tired, unable to concentrate, dizzy and overweight. Generally speaking, symptoms will worsen if salt intake is reduced and sometimes, if salt intake is increased, it will help to alleviate them.

The regulation of sodium depends largely on a healthy pair of adrenals. During mental or physical stress, adrenal activity changes markedly (see chapter on Stress). For example, during the course of an infection (latent viruses are a common cause of chronic fatigue), considerable demands are made upon the adrenal glands.

The amount of hormones stored in adrenal tissue are sufficient for only a few minutes in the absence of continual synthesis. For this reason, the rate of synthesis is extremely important to the rate of secretion.

Sodium deficiencies are among the most common endocrine disorders in clinical medicine. Failure to initiate salt-balance corrections may result in heart problems.

Sodium deficiencies make the body respond via the adrenals and their outpourings cause blood vessels to constrict, which results in poor oxygenation and reduced removal of waste products (such as lactic acid) from the blood. Lactic acid is what causes the muscular aches which sometimes follow exceptionally strenuous and prolonged muscular activity. An increase of lactate (the ionic form of lactic acid) can make muscles ache and cause anxiety in susceptible individuals.

Not surprisingly, excessive lactate is also a suspected cause of the muscular problems experienced by sufferers of chronic fatigue syndrome. In addition, many of the 'nerve' problems associated with chronic fatigue syndrome, such as anxiety, fearfulness, tension and irritability, can also be caused by excessive levels of lactate in the bloodstream. This type of anxiety is known as lactate induced anxiety syndrome (LIAS) and is discussed in the chapter on mood swings.

Cholesterol and liver functions

Nowadays, many people also endeavour to lower their cholesterol levels. Unfortunately, too little cholesterol can be just as bad as too much.

What most of us don't realise is that cholesterol is one of the ways in which the body disposes of some chemicals, notably mercury, and that many toxic chemicals are actually stored in fat.

Cholesterol is also an important source of adrenal hormones. The adrenals are usually filled with cholesterol which is transformed (biosynthesis) into adrenaline in the presence of Vitamin C. If we run short of these hormones because of a shortage of cholesterol, adrenal insufficiency may occur.

A sudden or excessive reduction in cholesterol could cause a lowering of blood pressure and swelling of the tissues with salt and water. The liver manufactures cholesterol and controls its levels in the blood.

When you are under stress, the body, in its wisdom, tells your liver to make more cholesterol so that the adrenals have enough to manufacture the extra stress hormones you need. This is one of the reasons why some people have increased levels of cholesterol when they are under stress, even though they may be following a low-cholesterol diet.

When we are exposed to foreign chemicals, an already bad situation is made worse because the liver has to work even harder to detoxify our system and to manufacture cholesterol. Many of the pathways used in the detoxification process are shared by alcohol and chemicals for which the liver is responsible.

Muscular weakness and aches

Many people who suffer with chronic fatigue also have problems with muscular weakness and aches. The adrenal cortex has a powerful and direct influence on muscle responses.

If we look at the classic disease involving impaired adrenal functions (Addison's disease), we see that among its symptoms are poor concentration, poor memory, drowsiness, depression, insomnia, restlessness, apprehension or anxiety, irritability, headaches, temporary blurring of vision, dizziness and tinnitus (ringing in the ears).

All those symptoms are also common in most people who suffer with chronic and unexplained fatigue. This, of course, does not imply that if you are unusually tired, or even if you are more tired than usual, and somewhat depressed, that you are a victim of chronic fatigue syndrome or suffer from Addison's disease.

However, we must question the possibility that many chronic fatigue sufferers exhibit a degree of adrenal insufficiency. Perhaps then we may find a surprisingly high incidence of sub-clinical hypoadrenocorticism among them.

How to improve adrenal functions

Worn-out adrenal glands can be helped by oral supplements of Vitamin B_5 (also known as calcium pantothenate or pantothenic acid, and found naturally in offal, eggs, wheat germ and royal jelly), liquorice, glycyrrhiza, sodium (salt), and a high protein diet that is not excessively low in cholesterol.

Vitamin C plays an important role not only in maintaining the adrenals' integrity, but in helping the conversion of cholesterol to adrenal hormones.

Other important nutrients are Vitamin A, Vitamin B_2 (riboflavin), zinc, magnesium and the amino acid tyrosine which requires both Vitamin C and calcium for its utilisation.

The tonic Korean (panax) ginseng, and herbs such as safflower, parsley, sarsaparilla, kelp, sage and savory also tend to help adrenal functions. A daily dose of garlic and sesame butter is also beneficial.

Foods high in Vitamin B_5 (pantothenic acid)

avocado	lobster
bean sprouts	mackerel
beef	mushrooms
chicken	peanuts
clams	pineapple
crab	salmon
egg	sardines
haddock	soya bean
lentils	watermelon
liver (beef, pork)	wheat germ

(Cont.)

(Cont.)

Foods high in Vitamin C (ascorbic acid)

alfalfa

banana

berries (blueberries, gooseberries, raspberries and strawberries)

Brazil nuts

broccoli

brussels sprouts

cabbage

cantaloupe melon

capsicum

cauliflower

citrus fruit (lemons, oranges, tomatoes)

guava

kidney

liver (beef)

oysters

potato

spinach

sweet potato

vegetables (green leafy ones)

watermelon

Foods high in Vitamin A

butter

carrots

crab

cream cheese

egg

grapefruit

halibut

liver (beef, fish)

margarine

melons

milk

oysters

salmon

spinach

squash

sweet potato

swordfish

tomato

vegetables (dark green, leafy ones)

Note that liquorice and glycyrrhiza are contraindicated in cases of high blood pressure, potassium deficiency and kidney disease, and that they also have a laxative effect.

Korean ginseng is also contraindicated in some cases of female hormonal and gynaecological problems, such as menorrhagia (abnormal bleeding from the uterus).

Tyrosine can aggravate some psychiatric disorders and is contraindicated in cases of melanoma cancer and in immune dysfunctions where the natural killer cells (NK) are low.

How to assess adrenal insufficiency

One of the simplest ways of assessing the possibility of adrenal insufficiency is to measure the blood pressure while the patient has been lying down relaxed or comfortably sitting down for a few minutes, and then immediately after the patient has moved quickly to a standing position.

The systolic pressure should be higher when the patient stands up suddenly. If it fails to increase or, worse still, if it decreases, then it indicates the possibility of adrenal impairment. The degree by which systolic blood pressure drops when in the standing position gives the therapist a rough estimate as to the degree of adrenal insufficiency.

Foods high in zinc

beef	mushrooms
bran	oatmeal
Brazil nuts	oysters
crab	pork
egg	pumpkin seeds
grains	rice, brown
herring	sunflower seeds
kidney	tuna
lamb	veal
milk	yeast (Brewer's)

Foods high in magnesium

almonds	beef
apricots, dried	Brazil nuts
avocado	carrots (raw)
baked beans	cashews
barley	chicken

(Cont.)

Food high in magnesium (Cont.)

citrus fruits	peas
corn	pecans
crab	pork
dates	potato
fish (flounder, salmon, tuna)	rice
lentils	sesame
Lima beans	soya beans
molasses	tomato (raw)
oatmeal	vegetables (dark green,
peaches	leafy ones)
peanuts	wheat germ

Another, more elaborate, method is the 'water loading' test and this can be carried out at home with simple instructions from a therapist, who should then interpret the results. This test is contraindicated in people with known kidney diseases.

Foods high in Vitamin B_2 (riboflavin)

almonds	flour
beans	mackerel
beef (kidney, heart, liver)	milk
blackcurrants	mushrooms
Brazil nuts	oysters
cheese	perch
chicken (liver)	rice
clams	salmon
cod	spinach
collard/kale	trout
egg	

5

AGEING AND ALZHEIMER'S DISEASE

'We begin to die the day we are born' is a rather unpalatable truism; however, growing old does not necessarily mean becoming senile. In fact, senility may well be somewhat of a myth according to some scientists who study the ageing process.

Until recently, symptoms such as memory loss, difficulties with bowel control, getting dressed or driving a car were considered a natural consequence of ageing. Today, this view has been discarded by the scientific community. Even at eighty, a decline in mental capacity is thought of as a disease, not a natural occurrence.

As we increase our life span, afflictions which were once rare have now become common. At the beginning of the 21st century about 16 per cent of the UK's population consisted of people aged over sixty-five and this figure is set to grow. According to the organisation Age Concern, the number of people aged ninety or over will increase by 50 per cent between 1996 and 2016. Senile dementia now affects one in twenty people over the age of seventy-five and one in five over the age of eighty.

Alzheimer's disease—diagnosis

Alzheimer's disease has been called 'the quiet epidemic', 'the silent disease' and 'the funeral that never ends'. By whatever name, the disastrous effects it has on its victims has been aptly described as a total destruction of the individual.

Senile dementia is the overall term given to many different diseases producing dementia. Over 50 per cent of dementia cases are considered to be sufferers of Alzheimer's disease. The Alzheimer's Society estimates that there are currently over 700,000 people in the UK with senile dementia.

The disease was first identified in 1906 by the German physician Alois Alzheimer. After the death of one of his patients, a 51-year-old woman with severe memory loss and mental confusion, Dr Alzheimer decided to conduct an autopsy on her brain and found the two distinctive characteristics of the disease: tangled lumps of brain nerve fibres and pockets of disintegrated nerve-cell branches.

There is a popular misconception that Alzheimer's disease can be readily diagnosed by its symptoms. However, this is not so and even now, the only way to be absolutely certain is to examine the brain after death.

The structural changes in the brain can be clearly seen with a low-powered microscope and seem to be concentrated in the cerebral cortex (where thought processes originate) and the hippocampus (which plays a special role in learning and memory processes).

Diagnosis while the patient is still alive remains largely a process of elimination. If, after a battery of tests, a physician can exclude strokes, Parkinson's disease, alcoholism, arteriosclerosis of the brain, tumours, depression, adverse drug reactions and side effects, or psychiatric problems, then the diagnosis is made by default.

There are other causes of dementia, notably multiple brain infarcts (a series of small strokes within the brain) and alcoholism. The disease would be easier to detect, and treat, if we knew exactly what causes it.

Another popular misconception about Alzheimer's disease is that certain signs, such as loss of memory, are the only, or at least sure; indications of the disease. Unfortunately, both the onset and progress of Alzheimer's disease are so insidious that they often escape recognition for months and even years. In addition, the early symptoms are varied and not easy to detect.

Consider the following. A woman can't remember whether she turned off the stove or locked the front door. A son noticed that his mother was not able to balance her chequebook and count change at the local grocery store. A businessman noticed that his wife uncharacteristically starts to indulge in wild spending sprees and is unable to make sense of simple phone messages. The wife of a handyman noticed a deterioration in her husband's quality of workmanship when walls were unevenly painted and a set of wall cabinets was so crooked no door would shut properly. Such aberrations are the marks which often signal the onset of Alzheimer's disease.

STAGES OF ALZHEIMER'S DISEASE

Age—abilities acquired	Disease stage—abilities lost
15+ get and hold a job	**Borderline** hold job
7–12 handle money	**Early stages** simple finances
5–7 select proper clothes	**Early stages** select clothes
5 years old put on clothes	**Moderate stage** put on clothes
4 years old go to toilet alone	**Severe** go to toilet alone
4 years old shower unaided	**Severe** shower unaided
2–3 years control bladder	**Late** control bladder
2–3 years control bowels	**Late** just control bowels
15 months speak a few words	**Late** just speak a few words
1 year speak one word	**Late stage** speak one word
1 year walk	**Late stage** walk
6–9 months sit up unaided	**Late stage** barely sit up unaided
2–3 months smile	**Late stage** smile

Is aluminium a cause of Alzheimer's disease? Are low levels of certain neurotransmitters the result of a systems failure which then produces the disease, or does Alzheimer's disease cause such failures and/or low levels of brain chemicals? Could the fault lie in altered patterns of receptors which then fail to respond adequately to neurotransmitters? Is it that a deficiency of some essential metal, such as calcium, magnesium or manganese, is suspected of allowing aluminium and perhaps other brain toxins to accumulate in the brain?

Or are there other factors, such as viral diseases, which disrupt natural protective mechanisms and allow the passage of toxic metals into the brain, across the so-called blood-brain barrier? Let us look at some of the current theories, hypotheses and ideas about Alzheimer's disease.

Heredity

Heredity may play a role because Alzheimer's disease often occurs in members of the same family. A sibling of an Alzheimer's disease sufferer has a 50 per cent chance of developing the disease, if they live long enough for the symptoms to manifest. Perhaps its onset is influenced or triggered by several genes so that anyone carrying them would only become a sufferer if they all combined simultaneously.

Apart from the statistical evidence, some scientists believe that because almost all Down's syndrome sufferers develop Alzheimer's disease by the age of forty, there is a strong heredity factor. So strongly do some medical scientists believe in this theory that at least one doctor claims he has found a way with nutritional therapy to prevent Alzheimer's disease and in some cases even reverse some of its effects.

Dr Chris Reading, a Sydney psychiatrist who is widely recognised as Australia's pioneer of nutritional psychiatry, is also an expert in human genetics and believes he has found a link between illnesses such as leukaemia, Alzheimer's disease, Down's syndrome and schizophrenia. 'These diseases often occur over several generations of the same family and appear to have similar causes', says Dr Reading.

His success with sufferers of Alzheimer's disease stems from his work with Down's syndrome children. After testing four thousand patients over a six-year period, Dr Reading discovered that some vitamin and mineral deficiencies as well as inherited food or chemical allergies or intolerances cause abnormal growths, and the development of Alzheimer's disease in children with Down's syndrome.

If their nutritional problems and allergies are treated in time, there is a strong likelihood that they will not develop Alzheimer's disease in later years. Dr Reading is currently working to assess if such preventive measures may apply to other susceptible individuals and perhaps to the general population.

Viruses

Knowing that many Alzheimer's disease sufferers seldom appear 'ill' and hardly ever show signs of infection, such as a fever or elevated white cell count, it seems strange that anyone should consider viral infections as a possible cause.

However, some scientists speculate that one of the 'slow' or 'retro' viruses may be responsible. Since the discovery, in the 1960s, of viruses which are capable of causing harm years after the original infection has taken place, we have come to realise that it is possible a viral agent may cause Alzheimer's disease and perhaps several other diseases for which we have no explanation at present.

The possibility exists that a virus may impair the activity or synthesis of key brain enzymes or even neurotransmitters.

Abnormal proteins

There is little doubt that Alzheimer's disease is associated with protein abnormalities. The nerve cells tangle and complex proteins (which resemble starch (amyloids)) surround and invade both cerebral blood vessels and degenerating nerve endings.

These are characteristic findings in Alzheimer's disease but so far nobody has been able to say if they are the cause or the effect of the disease. Indeed, the possibility exists that, if they are abnormal, the synthesis of the proteins could be dictated by abnormal genes, making it an hereditary or genetic abnormality.

It may also be possible that abnormal or defective enzymes are activated by environmental toxins and then these enzymes synthesise modified proteins which choke, as it were, normal brain cells. These protein bundles, called neurofibrillary tangles, are numerous in the brain stem neurons which release neurotransmitters in general and acetylcholine in particular.

The amyloids tend to collect in the middle layers of blood vessels in the brain and advance outward where they eventually weaken and even replace the walls. This weakening of the blood-vessel walls may explain the local haemorrhages which are common in the last stages of Alzheimer's disease.

Local haemorrhages are technically known as strokes. Repeated small cerebral strokes can give rise to the same symptoms as someone suffering late stage Alzheimer's disease. It is often difficult to know, until after death, if the patient is suffering from true Alzheimer's disease.

Neurotransmitters

Neurotransmitters are natural chemicals which the brain makes from common amino acids. These are the basic constituents of proteins derived from the food we eat every day.

Neurotransmitters are substances which enable brain cells to communicate with each other. They are, in other words, chemical messengers within the brain and central nervous system.

While each neurotransmitter has a specific function in the brain, most have more than one and, in almost all cases, the quantity of each is not always as important as the ratio between two or more of them at any one time. Even if one allows that Alzheimer's disease needs a combination of factors to occur, the fact remains that one or more neurotransmitters are linked with the disease.

In the mid-1970s Dr Peter Davies, then at the Institute of Neurology in London, showed that the brains of people with Alzheimer's disease contained drastically reduced levels (up to 90 per cent) of a key enzyme, choline acetyltransferase (CAT). This enzyme is needed by the brain to produce a chemical neurotransmitter known as acetylcholine which is made from the amino acid choline and acetyl coenzyme A (requiring Vitamin B_1 and Vitamin B_5).

When David Drachman of the University of Massachusetts Medical Centre administered a drug called Scopolamine (known to interfere with acetylcholine memory mechanisms), the temporary state of mental confusion and memory loss was virtually indistinguishable from that of someone with Alzheimer's disease. This supports the theory that memory impairment is associated with a decrease in acetylcholine levels.

Experiments calculated to increase. levels of CAT enzymes, or to reduce the rate of acetylcholine breakdown, have shown that the

Foods high in choline

bean sprouts	liver (beef, pork)
beef	milk
chickpeas	peanuts
egg yolk	split peas
green beans	soy
lentils	

rate at which the neurotransmitter is synthesised is not necessarily limited by the amount of enzymes but by the availability of the precursor substances from which acetylcholine is manufactured, namely choline and acetyl coenzyme A.

Giving patients large amounts of choline or lecithin as a supplement has shown that it does help to reduce the symptoms of Alzheimer's disease. A carefully controlled study by Raymond Levy of the University of London Faculty of Medicine found continuing behavioural improvements in eight out of twenty-four patients treated in this way. While encouraging, results such as these strongly suggest that there are several forms of Alzheimer's disease.

Because autopsies of Alzheimer's disease sufferers reveal physical destruction of nerve cell terminals, it is also possible that, when faced with a shortage of choline from which to synthesise acetylcholine, the brain cannibalises some of its own cell membranes for their content of phosphatidlycholine (a ready source of choline).

Other neurotransmitters may be implicated. Norepinephrine and serotonin seem to be lacking in the brains of patients with Alzheimer's disease (*New Scientist*, June 1985, p. 34) and the level of glutamate in the cerebrospinal fluid correlates with the severity of the dementia.

The neurotransmitter hypothesis does not preclude that of environmental toxins or nutrient (other than choline, Vitamin B_1 and Vitamin B_5) deficiencies because toxins such as aluminium may well block neurotransmitters, their synthesis or perhaps their activity.

The complex interactions of nutrients, such as vitamins and minerals, also make it possible that a specific deficiency of one of these may upset the delicate balance between neurotransmitters, their precursors or the enzymes necessary for their synthesis.

Environmental deficiencies

Many people like to blame our deteriorating environment, particularly the chemicalisation of air, water and food supplies, for almost all our health problems, while others are convinced that deficiencies of various nutrients, especially vitamins and minerals, are at the root of all modern diseases.

However, these two factors very often interact in ways that cause, or at least trigger, many illnesses. Where an individual is susceptible, either because of an inherent trait or because of heredity, any factor may well precipitate Alzheimer's disease without anyone being able to *prove* a direct cause-and-effect relationship.

We know, for example, that people who smoke more than one packet of cigarettes per day are four times more likely to get Alzheimer's disease than non-smokers; yet no one is suggesting tobacco *causes* Alzheimer's disease. Many environmental factors exist which may trigger, aggravate or cause Alzheimer's disease.

Consider the following. In the remote Pacific island of Guam, there is a tribe known as the Chamarros whose members suffer from a high incidence of amyotrophic lateral sclerosis (ALS) which causes progressive muscular wasting, Parkinson's disease-like tremors, Alzheimer's disease-like dementia and neuron tangles. It just so happens that the area of Guam in which the Chamarros live is almost totally deficient in magnesium and calcium. We already know that a deficiency of calcium (or of Vitamin D_3) tends to favour the accumulation of strontium 90, aluminium and perhaps several other toxic metals.

Neuropathologist, Dr Daniel Perl, of the University of Vermont College of Medicine, believes that the deficits of magnesium and calcium combined with the accumulation of heavy metals such as aluminium may play a role in the beginning of Alzheimer's disease.

Diuretics (water pills) are taken by millions of people in an effort to reduce high blood pressure and prevent heart disease. These drugs tend to increase the loss of several minerals such as calcium, magnesium, zinc and other essential micronutrients through the

SOME COMMON, AND NOT SO COMMON, SOURCES OF ALUMINIUM

Aluminium cookware including utensils

The following list outlines problems with cooking in aluminium:

- boiling water produces hydro-oxides, which are toxic
- boiling eggs produces phosphates, which inhibit the absorption of calcium
- boiling meat produces chlorides
- frying bacon increases nitrates
- vegetables tend to produce neutralising factors which impede proper digestion of food
- teapots are particularly suspect because the tannic acid in tea tends to allow aluminium to leak into the beverage

Water supplies

- special chemicals, called flocculating agents, are used in water purification (sic!)
- hot water pipes are sometimes made with cathodic corrosion preventatives which are made from aluminium

Food additives

Aluminium is a common food additive in foods such as:

- cheese, table salt, baking powders, pickles, maraschino cherries, vanilla powders and bleached flours
- even milk formulae for babies contain up to four hundred times more aluminium than that found in breast milk

General additives

- toothpastes
- nasal sprays
- anti-perspirants
- dental amalgams
- cigarette filters
- aspirin compounds
- pesticides (which also end up as residue in some foodstuffs)

urinary system. Many people already have marginal levels of these nutrients and may not be left with enough to prevent toxic metals, such as aluminium, from accumulating in their brains.

Dr Perl has also shown that the tangled nerve fibres in the brains of people suffering from Alzheimer's disease contain unusually large amounts of aluminium and that this metal, when injected into the brains of animals, leads to similar deterioration. His research suggests that aluminium accumulates preferentially in brain cells.

Other researchers, such as Donald Maclaughlin of the University of Toronto Faculty of Medicine, have shown that neuron tangles will develop in the brains of experimental animals when aluminium salts are injected.

Irreversible dementia is seen in some people who have undergone kidney dialyses with aluminium-rich solutions. In addition, we know that aluminium salts can inhibit some key brain enzymes as well as the transport of essential proteins. (*Scientific American*, Jan. 1985, p. 48).

The possible involvement of aluminium in Alzheimer's disease was discussed widely at the Royal Society meeting in London (April 1987) and several scientists proposed that, quite apart from the obvious sources of this metal (see list on page 107), acid rain may be a major culprit. Aluminium is known to be the toxin responsible for the death of fish in streams and lakes rendered acid by polluted rain. Aluminium dissolves in these waters instead of silicon: aluminium is toxic to humans, while silicon is essential for life.

Aluminium is the third most common element on earth, after oxygen and silicon, and the most prevalent metal in the crust of our planet. It is, therefore, not easy to avoid but this is no reason to use antacids, deodorants, baking powders and aluminium cookware—not to mention aluminium in one's tap or rain water. The best solution for the latter seems to be using a good quality water filter. There is aluminium foil, aluminium cans and even airconditioning bombards us with aluminium particles from their cooling units.

There is still much debate as to whether the aluminium concentration is a cause or an effect of Alzheimer's disease. It is, however, possible that aluminium may cause the problem indirectly.

According to a study by Banks and Atkins of the Veterans Administration Medical Center and Department of Medicine at

Tulane University School of Medicine in New Orleans, aluminium may alter the permeability of the natural barrier which protects the brain from unwanted substances: the blood-brain barrier (*The Lancet* ii, 1983: 1227–1229).

It is speculated that this change in the permeability of the blood-brain barrier may allow other environmental toxins, and perhaps inimical proteins, to enter the brain and alter its functions. We already have a tentative model for this in the case of epilepsy which can be triggered, if not caused, by excessive amounts of the otherwise harmless, even essential, vitamin factor, folic acid, leaking, as it were, into the brain of people prone to seizures.

Apart from the fact that aluminium is ubiquitous, there is the problem with absorption: this toxic metal can be readily absorbed into the body through the gastrointestinal tract (*New England Journal of Medicine* No. 310(17), 107).

Not many Britons realise that the sale of aluminium cookware is prohibited in Germany, France, Switzerland, Belgium, Hungary and Brazil.

Alcohol

According to Alcohol Concern, the national agency on alcohol misuse, one person in thirteen in Britain is dependent on alcohol—twice as many as are addicted to all sorts of drugs, including prescription drugs. To what extent long-term drinking affects the brain and how many cases of senility and Alzheimer's disease are, in fact, the result of the adverse effects of alcohol, is anyone's guess.

Alcohol exerts a powerful influence on the human brain. It stimulates the production of brain chemicals (endorphins) which act as an anaesthetic. It dulls physical pain and also depresses those centres in the brain which are responsible for controlling behaviour and co-ordination. Alcohol irritates the gut linings and can be responsible for malabsorption of nutrients essential for brain functions.

After all, almost without exception, every chemical (neurotransmitter) used by the brain is made from a food-derived amino acid and its synthesis requires the presence and co-ordination of several vitamins, minerals and other essential nutrients.

This is evident from the fact that many neurological disorders are caused directly by a deficiency of Vitamin B_1 (thiamine), which is a state caused by alcoholism. Professor Byron Kakulas, head of Neuropathology at Royal Perth Hospital, claims that many of the effects of alcohol on the brain can be nullified by taking a few vitamins, especially Vitamin B_1, which would immediately reduce some of the most common mental disorders associated with alcohol abuse. It should also be noted that Vitamin B_1 is essential for one of the key biochemical steps in which acetylcholine (a brain neurotransmitter associated with Alzheimer's disease) is synthesised from the amino acid choline.

Foods high in Vitamin B_1 (thiamine)

beef (heart, liver, kidney)	pork (liver)
Brazil nuts	poultry
cereals	pumpkin
fish (mackerel,	soya bean
perch, red snapper)	sunflower seeds
lamb	wheat
milk	wheat germ
oatmeal	yeast (Brewer's)
peas and other legumes	

Blood sugar

We have become so involved with the problems of hypoglycaemia (low or fluctuating blood sugar) that we tend to forget some of the devastating effects that high blood-sugar (glucose) levels can cause.

We have long known that diabetics tend to be prone to infections and that their susceptibility is influenced by how well the disease (or blood-sugar level) is controlled. We also know that several of the complications of diabetes mimic the degenerative processes of old age; in particular, senile cataracts, joint stiffness and atherosclerosis develop earlier in diabetics.

Collagen, the most abundant extra-cellular protein that glues cells together, degenerates when it is exposed to glucose. Blood sugar, in other words, may well play a role in the tissue changes associated with degenerative processes such as old age. We do not know at this stage if these changes extend to, or are able to influence, brain cells, but it gives people another good reason not to eat excessive amounts of sweets.

This, you may think, exonerates hypoglycaemia (low blood sugar) as even a circumstantial culprit in Alzheimer's disease. Unfortunately, this is not so.

The blood flow-hypoglycaemia-hypoxia hypothesis

My grandparents used to blame almost everything on 'poor circulation' and chiropractors know only too well how many health problems can be relieved or cured by manipulations calculated to increase circulation in general, and blood flow to specific areas.

The normal blood flow to the brain tends to diminish by about 20 per cent between the early thirties and sixties but the brain compensates for this by extracting proportionally more oxygen from it.

In Alzheimer's disease blood flow diminishes more than average and the associated compensatory uptake of oxygen does not happen. Both the blood flow and oxygen consumption continue to decline in parallel as the clinical picture of someone suffering from Alzheimer's disease deteriorates.

Dr Frank Benson of the University of California at Los Angeles School of Medicine found that as little as half the normal amounts of glucose were consumed by the brains of those with Alzheimer's disease. Glucose provides brain cells with all their energy requirements; however, this is only possible if oxygen is available at the same time.

Other researchers have found that levels of special enzymes needed to convert glucose to energy are deficient in brain samples of people affected by Alzheimer's disease. Can these factors be influenced by regular chiropractic treatment, exercise, good diet and a healthy lifestyle? Common sense would say so.

A FEW TIPS

As old age approaches, what can *you* do to avoid, or at least try to prevent, becoming a victim of Alzheimer's disease? Here are a few tips:

1. Make sure your blood-sugar levels are normal and under control. A glucose tolerance test (GTT) is one way to be sure. If there is a history of diabetes in your family, then these checks should be done periodically. In general, though, it is advisable to avoid excessive sugars, sweets and refined carbohydrates as well as alcohol.
2. If you have the faintest suspicion that you are allergic/intolerant to anything, be it food, chemicals or inhalants, have someone check this out and arrange prompt treatment.
3. Avoid, as far as humanly possible, all additives, colourants, pesticides, toxic chemicals and pollution sources.
4. Unless absolutely necessary, do not use drugs or medicines that will negatively affect your blood flow, amino acid utilisation or absorption, brain function, mineral and vitamin absorption or metabolism. If you **have** to take some medicines, make sure you also take the appropriate vitamins, essential nutrients and mineral supplements to compensate for this.
5. Do all you can to avoid succumbing to viral infections. At the very least, this means taking daily supplements of a strong Vitamin C plus zinc compound.
6. Make sure your body is getting the best from foods you eat by ensuring that your digestive system is performing well. This may mean supplementary hydrochloric acid and biotin, especially if you are over fifty, and digestive enzymes. Remember also that some protein foods, such as eggs and fish, may actually enhance brain functions in old age.
7. Take choline supplements (in lecithin form) and never go short of Vitamin B_1 and Vitamin B_5, especially if you drink alcohol or eat lots of sweets and refined carbohydrates.

(Cont.)

A Few Tips (Cont.)

8. Make sure you get enough calcium, magnesium and Vitamin D_3, especially so if you are exposed to aluminium.

9. Avoid aluminium as far as humanly possible. Drink from glass containers and wrap your food in plain oiled paper.

10. Use a good water filter.

11. Drink moderate amounts of alcohol only **with** meals.

12. Get plenty of exercise and fresh air to ensure good circulation.

13. Vitamin E and niacin help blood flow, so take some every day.

14. Have regular chiropractic or osteopathic adjustments as blood flow through your body and to your brain, in particular, may be drastically affected by unknown subluxations.

6

STRESS

People everywhere suffer from stress. Doctors prescribe tranquillisers for it, politicians retire because of it and mystics teach ways to try to overcome it. We are all subjected to stress.

However, as bad as we may think it is, stress is also an essential process that keeps our adrenal glands working. When stress is too much, however, a potentially dangerous situation arises. Our metabolism is unable to cope and adjust and this paves the way for various illnesses, degenerative diseases and emotional problems.

Stress is activated by many factors and, in order to cope, we must be able to recognise the symptoms and have at our disposal a kitbag full of resources to correct stress-induced imbalances.

What is stress?

What is stress? The man who invented the concept, Dr Hans Selye, Professor and Director of the Institute of Experimental Medicine and Surgery at the University of Montreal, Canada, who also holds doctorates in medicine, science and philosophy, gives this definition in his book *Stress Without Distress*:

Everybody knows what stress is, and nobody knows what it is. The word stress, like success, failure or happiness, means different things to different people and, except for a few specialised scientists, no-one has really tried to define it, although it has become part of our everyday vocabulary.

If the weather suddenly turns cold and windy, you are likely to shiver. If it gets hot, you'll sweat. If you eat too much sugar, your body will react by pumping out hormones which will cause it to be stored or burned. Run uphill and your heart will race faster. If you are in pain, if you are lonely or if you lose too much blood from an injury, you experience stress.

While the mechanism of stress (called the non-specific response) is the same for all of us, the particular way in which each of us reacts to stress is different. In fact, one may react in different ways to the same stress at different times. To paraphrase Hippocrates, 'One man's stress is another man's ecstasy'. Let's face it, some people yearn to be whipped while others faint at the sight of blood.

Our ancestors lived precarious lives where each day was a stressful challenge just to find enough food to stay alive. Why, then, is it more of a problem these days? The answer lies in the fact that primitive man always took some physical action in response to stress and, in so doing, got it out of their system—they either killed the wild beasts, or were killed by them. The physical action necessary to combat stress, the 'fight or flight' response, burned up energy, cholesterol, superfluous hormones and, after a while, things returned to normal.

People are subjected to many different stresses every day but, unlike our ancestors, there is nowhere to run or nothing to attack—you just sit feeling sick and fuming under the action of powerful hormones. Enough of these events, and sooner or later the body or the mind is unable to cope and breaks down. This is called psychosomatic or psychogenic illness.

However, it should also be remembered that there are different types of stress and that not all stress is bad for you. Take, for example, events such as getting married, concluding a business deal, or winning a competitive event; all these are forms of stress. However, if you avoided all stress, which is impossible, you might live a little longer but you might also die of boredom!

How does stress affect your body?

Dr Selye defines stress as 'the non-specific response of the body to any demands made upon it'. The key word here is non-specific, and it is these responses that can't be seen. You *can*, however, see the obvious *specific* effects of some of the non-specific responses, for example crying, fainting, shivering, sweating, vomiting. All these are individual responses: they vary from time to time, and from person to person. Sometimes people can adjust to some stresses so that they no longer react to them in a particular way. You may break out in a cold sweat the first time you fly, but after a few times you gradually adjust to it.

The non-specific responses are those which are going on off-camera—down in the engine room, so to speak. The non-specific response causes the specific response in order to make the body adjust to the situation. If you get cold enough, you'll shiver, shivering is motion and motion creates heat, and so the body temperature rises.

The body has 'adjusted'. In order to understand how the body adjusts to non-specific responses it helps to know something about the production of hormones secreted by the endocrine system.

The adrenal glands sit on top of each kidney, and produce the hormone adrenaline. Aggression, drive and energy are what we associate with adrenalin. However, the adrenals are under the rule of a little gland that sits at the base of the skull, called the pituitary, and this gland is controlled by the hypothalamus.

The hypothalamus is a pocket, or ventricle, in the brain which acts as a monitoring device on all incoming messages from outside and from inside the body—sound, taste, smell, blood pressure, acidity, fluid concentrations in the blood, and so on. The hypothalamus is also called the 'neuroendrocrinal transducer' because it translates (transduces) messages from nerve-impulses into endocrinal (hormonal) messages.

These messages are translated into chemicals called releasing factors, hormone-like substances that travel down a little stalk connected to the pituitary, and cause it to send off releasing hormones. The adrenals get some of these chemical messages (as well as others from the autonomic nervous system), and the alarm bell goes off!

Whether the alarm is caused by an enzyme in distress because we've eaten foods we can't cope with, or because we hear the baby crying, the adrenaline pours out into the bloodstream. Once this happens, the heart pumps faster, blood pressure rises, air passages enlarge, blood is drawn from the skin to muscles (now you know why your face becomes white with fear) and digestion is interrupted.

The blood, full of adrenaline, then reaches the pituitary, and causes more hormones to shoot down to the other half of the adrenals, causing them to start pumping out some of their many hormones. Meantime, the thyroid, para-thyroid, pancreas and sex glands begin to secrete some of their particular hormones too.

The result of this biochemical sleight-of-hand is to send little shock waves into just about every corner of your body, revving it up, as it were, for action. However, too often nowadays, the strenuous action that makes use of all these functions does not follow.

Major substances released by the adrenals are the glucocorticoids, which increase blood-sugar levels so more energy is available. In response to this, the pancreas must then secrete insulin to bring blood-sugar levels down again when all the excitement is over. So even a candy bar or excess sugar can act as a form of stress.

Not only does the pancreas resent having to deal with an extra sudden rise in blood sugar but, if it happens too often, it may over-react so violently that blood-sugar levels fall too much. The body then has to create more blood sugar—often out of body proteins—or more sugar has to be eaten. And so the vicious circle starts all over again and the body is then in the constant grip of biochemical stress. This last example is a form of hypoglycaemia.

The adrenals also secrete cortisone, which dulls the body's immune response. You get a cold, 'flu and other infections more easily when you are over-stressed.

The thyroid is also affected and tells the body to increase its metabolic rate. This means that fat stores are raided to make extra energy, body proteins are also sometimes broken down, calcium is leached from the bones, vitamins are used up more quickly and the gastro-intestinal tract races overtime, sometimes producing diarrhoea. So when you are still huffing and fuming hours (even days) after the stressful event, the situation gets serious.

STRESS CONCEPT OF DISEASE

Dr Selye put all the assorted miseries of the endocrine system into a neat package, which he called the 'Stress Concept of Disease'.

During experiments in which he was injecting rats with different substances, he noticed that all the animals developed enlarged adrenal glands (a sure sign of overwork), their thymus, spleen and lymph nodes shrank, and they developed ulcers.

Eventually, he discovered that practically all toxic substances, whether chemicals or drugs, could cause practically the same effects. Looking at humans, Dr Selye found that these responses occurred in all kinds of patients, whether suffering from cancer, infections or psychological stress.

If the mechanism is the same, why does stress affect different people in so many different ways, whereas the rats all got ulcers? Dr Selye proposed that this was because animals used in experiments tend to be of the same breed, the same age, even from the same litter. Whereas humans have environmental differences, hereditary weakness, different occupational stresses, different emotional reactions, and a great difference in nutritional status.

It's a question of where the weak link is. That is why tension at work will give one person high blood pressure, another an ulcer, and another a headache. Yet all these have one common factor—the alarm went off, and the endocrinal glands went to work pushing out their hormones.

The effects of stress are cumulative. In other words, they add up and constant little stresses can eventually produce greater health problems. Take noise, for example. It has been found that people living near airports or on flight-paths tend to have more illnesses, especially cardiovascular illness, than those who don't. Noise is a form of stress. Even though after a while you get used to it and don't notice it, the body's alarm bell still goes off every time a plane lands or takes off.

Over the years, the long-term effects of stress hormones pouring out at all odd hours of the day and night can produce disastrous results: immune responses are lowered, the kidneys and heart are overworked, blood pressure is on the up-and-up, diabetes is more likely (because glucocorticoids tend to elevate blood-sugar levels), and the pancreas is hard-pressed to keep up the extra supply of insulin needed.

Stress and the food you eat

In our modern society, one of the most over-worked organs is the liver. This is because, among other things, it has to keep changing the molecules of foods that we eat into different ones—some for storage, some for tissue building and some for antibodies.

The liver also has to detoxify practically every foreign chemical we eat (antibiotics, colourings, preservatives), as well as excess fats, excess carbohydrates, excess proteins and all alcohol. And if all this is not enough, it also has to break down many hormones after they have carried out messages.

If we continually pile up more and more work on the liver—as we do every time we take a drug, eat too much of something, drink too much or inhale or ingest chemicals—its energy goes down. The liver then has less energy left to take care of 'alarm' hormones and so they remain in the blood stream longer than they should and their nasty side-effects accumulate.

So by eating over-refined, processed foods, we place our body under subtle but relentless stresses. While we are doing this, we are also depleting our stores of vitamins and other essential co-workers of our enzyme system. We place undue strain on the machinery of our body, and we become more and more susceptible to a whole range of diseases of the body and the mind.

There is no clear-cut, cause-and-effect correlation between what we eat and getting cancer, bronchitis or depression but you may well find that air pollution, food additives, plus an inability to adapt to or cope with some unhealthy foods, plus the stresses of modern life can all add up to illness. Everyone is biochemically unique: one man's meat can literally be another man's poison.

By following these simple steps you can avoid some of the every-day, in-built stresses that are placed on your body.

How to Avoid Stress by Mouth

1. Find out whether you are unsuited to a certain type of diet. Vegetarianism is considered a healthy diet. However, if you happen to be affected by natural compounds found in many fruits and vegetables, called salicylates, your choice of fruit and vegetables would be very restricted. Most nutritionists are able to arrange for tests to assess the suitability of any given diet.
2. Once you have established a diet that agrees with your metabolism then work out which foods within that dietary regime cause your body less stress. For example, you may know that you are sensitive to certain types of grains or that dairy foods cause you a problem, and so these should be avoided.
3. Try to avoid eating large amounts of refined and processed foods. If you are partial to certain foods that fall into this category, remember to give your body a break from these by eating fresh, simple foods to allow your body to recuperate.
4. Remember to supplement your diet with appropriate vitamins and minerals to help your enzymes function properly. An adequate supply of specific vitamins to suit your individual needs will also help your body to resist and withstand stress.

Strange isn't it, that everybody knows that working too hard or sleeping too little are both stresses that should be avoided or minimised whenever possible, but so few people stop to think that refined, processed foods with preservatives and additives are just as much a source of subtle but continuous biochemical stress on your body.

Let us imagine that health and stress are the scales of justice. On one side you have 'stress resistance' (50 grams) and on the other side you have 'unavoidable stresses' (50 grams). If your 'unavoidable stresses' are polluted air (10 grams), take-away foods (15 grams) and alcohol (10 grams), then you only have 15 grams left before you have tipped the scales beyond your stress resistance.

There are many people who seem to understand this credit and debit approach to health. It's not uncommon to find smokers who take more care of their diet and take special supplements to minimise the effects of smoking, or people who'll only eat dessert if they have faithfully stuck to their exercise schedule.

These people are not fooling themselves because little things do make a difference, and they have grasped the essential point: health is balance.

7

PREMENSTRUAL SYNDROME

When I was a young boy, women menstruated but *never* talked about it. However, nowadays the monthly period has become a subject that we can all talk about more freely. After all, if a condition such as premenstrual tension exists which makes your life and that of your partner unbearable, then it should be talked about and something should be done about it.

In the past, the best help that was offered was a tranquilliser and more often than not the unhappy sufferers were advised to take control of themselves. Nowadays there is a veritable cornucopia of premenstrual tension remedies, mostly in the form of nutritional supplements or herbs. Some of these do work for some women, some of the time. There are, however, reasons why it is difficult to treat all sufferers successfully.

We are now discovering that there are many different types of premenstrual syndromes (which should not surprise anybody considering that females are even more biochemically unique than males) which can be helped by different types and combinations of supplements and diets.

Research and the experience of clinical practice has shown that some of our patients will get better no matter what formula they take, while others will not. In many instances, I have noted that some of my patients actually get worse with certain types of supplements, especially those containing yeast, large amounts of folic acid and iron. The same applies to diets: while most women do benefit from avoiding fatty animal meats, some actually become worse if they switch to a complete vegetarian diet.

Premenstrual tension (PMT), as the syndrome is popularly referred to, can cause wild and uncontrollable mood swings and, in most cases, it *is* treatable provided the therapist can formulate a diet and supplements regimen that is suited to the individual.

SYMPTOMS OF PREMENSTRUAL TENSION

Psychological symptoms irritability, nervous tension, anxiety, mood swings, aggressiveness, fatigue, inability to dream, lack of sex drive, depression, poor memory, inability to think clearly and mental confusion, food cravings

Physical symptoms abdominal swelling, general increase in weight and fluid retention, headaches, swelling and tenderness of breasts, muscular weakness, body aches and pains.

Types of premenstrual syndrome

Specialists often divide premenstrual syndrome sufferers into five distinct subgroups. At the Complementary and Environmental Medicine Centre in Sydney, we have successfully treated many thousands of patients with premenstrual syndrome and recognised at least seven subgroups with varying symptoms for which a combination of dietary and supplementary treatments may be useful.

A CASE OF PREMENSTRUAL BLUES AND OTHER PROBLEMS

Sally walked into my office looking a picture of dejection. 'I am twenty-six years old and for at least one week every month I feel like I'm ninety-six! I become depressed, have incredible cravings for

(Cont.)

A Case of Premenstrual Blues (Cont.)

chocolate (which I binge on) and retain kilos of fluid. My skin gets ruined and it takes weeks before it starts to look presentable again. By then, my next period is due, and the whole thing starts again!'

I asked Sally about her past pregnancies and she told me that she had suffered with toxaemia both times. When I heard this I explained to her that Vitamin B_6 is reported to prevent and even cure toxaemia of pregnancy. Interestingly, the same vitamin also has a reputation for reducing premenstrual depression, anxiety and the flare-up of skin conditions associated with oestrogen sensitivities. It also exerts a diuretic effect and thus helps to reduce fluid retention.

So I prescribed Vitamin B_6 to be taken three times a day with meals. I also asked Sally to take Vitamin E because this nutrient is not only a useful antioxidant and circulation booster, but it also helps to counteract the effects of any excessive oestrogen. Next, I prescribed the oil of evening primrose, as this is known to reduce many of the stress symptoms associated with premenstrual syndrome, especially the mood swings. It does not, however, have any effect on oestrogen or fluid retention.

Sally started to protest, 'How many pills do you want me to take? I'll be so full I won't need to eat!' I told her, however, that this was not all as there were two aspects of her premenstrual syndrome that required special attention. She not only craved and binged on chocolate every month, which caused her to be constipated and aggravated her skin, but she also suffered a considerable amount of pain with her period.

There is a particular nutrient, actually an amino acid, called DL-phenylalanine (DLPA) which not only acts as a powerful yet natural painkiller, but is also a good antidepressant and stops most people from craving chocolate. (The reason is that chocolate contains a natural chemical, phenylethylalanine, which is converted to DLPA in the body.)

So it was natural for Sally to seek solace with chocolate and DLPA would do the same job without making her constipated or causing

(Cont.)

A Case of Premenstrual Blues (Cont.)

any worsening of her skin. I also added a Vitamin C formula to her regimen because her urine test showed practically no Vitamin C and this nutrient is a powerful antioxidant and a natural antihistamine.

I saw Sally again five weeks later and she looked, and apparently felt, like a new woman. 'I could not believe it,' she exclaimed. 'I hardly noticed my last period. It came on almost without any warning! My skin looks quite normal and I feel happy.'

1. PMS-T (tension)

Symptoms include nervous tension, irritability, anxiety, aggressiveness, anger, uncontrollable mood swings, palpitations, crying spells and tantrums, low libido.

While some of the symptoms may be associated with, and perhaps aggravated by, high oestrogen levels and a relative deficiency of progesterone, the most common contributing factors in PMS-T are excessive alcohol consumption, decreased liver function, the use of oral contraceptives, excessive consumption of sugars and refined carbohydrates, and a stressful lifestyle.

These patients appear to benefit from an intake of calcium (in the orotate form), Vitamin B_6, magnesium, zinc, ascorbic acid and a diet which contains a reasonable amount of proteins. Spirulina seems to be ideal for these patients. Oil of evening primrose can also help while Vitamin B_3 (pantothenic acid) can make them worse.

PMS-T patients are ideal candidates for hypnotherapy, counselling, biofeedback and other forms of relaxation-inducing, stress-lowering techniques.

We have also found that PMS-T sufferers tend to have elevated sensitivity to excess copper in their food or liquid intake. They often drink lots of tap water and use the hot-water tap to make tea and coffee which causes additional copper to be consumed. In addition to advising them on safer drinking techniques, such as the use of a water filter, zinc and Vitamin C supplements are particularly useful.

PREMENSTRUAL SYNDROME AND AGGRESSION

It has been estimated that 90 per cent of all aggressive behaviour in women occurs around the time of their menstrual period and nearly half of all crimes committed by females are perpetrated during menstruation or just before. More than half of the female population of Australia suffers from premenstrual syndrome.

---

2. PMS-E *(oestrogen)*

Symptoms include irritability, anxiety and most of the symptoms of PMS-T, breast swelling and tenderness, clotty menstrual blood, fluid retention.

PMS-E sufferers are diagnosed differently from PMS-T because of the likelihood that this condition is caused or aggravated by excessive oestrogen.

In many cases these women tend to have periodic food cravings, but not always for sweet substances. PMS-E women are often adversely affected by oral contraceptives (because the oestrogen content aggravates matters) and insufficient progesterone—a hormone that has been used with some success in the medical treatment of PMS.

Hypothyroidism goes hand in hand with increased oestrogen levels, so each patient has to be carefully examined for low-thyroid function.

Excessive oestrogen levels are also associated with heart disease and some forms of cancer. Carleton Frederick, author of *Breast Cancer*, suggests that breast tenderness and swelling and fluid retention may be aggravated by too much folic acid and para-amino-benzoic acid (PABA). Folic acid increases the effects of oestrogen and PABA can exacerbate some of its effects.

Some women on a high-vegetable, low-protein diet appear to have menstrual problems which are reversed when their intake of vegetables, especially carrots, is decreased. Apart from the fact that many vegetables are high in folic acid, and this could presumably affect susceptible females, carrots and other vegetables contain oestrogen-like substances.

OESTROGEN AND THE CALIFORNIAN DESERT QUAIL

Oestrogen acts as a natural contraceptive and the delicate balance required for this hormone can be seen by investigating the Californian Desert Quail.

When there is little rain, these birds appear to breed less. It now seems that during a drought, the seeds on which the quail feed produce additional oestrogen. This acts as a contraceptive and therefore the number of birds competing for the dwindling food supplies are reduced. When rain is abundant, the oestrogen content of the seeds is diluted and the bird population increases.

Many plants, such as clover, lucerne, rye grasses and soya, contain plant phenols or isoflavones which are substances known as phyto-oestrogens because they mimic the activity of the natural female hormone. The phyto-oestrogens are also present in cows' milk and are more prevalent in the skimmed variety favoured by so many these days.

PMS-E women should be given ample amounts of Vitamin B_6, magnesium and zinc but *not* B-complex formulas (which contain large amounts of folic acid), para-amino-benzoic acid, calcium pantothenate or calcium. Although Vitamin C is recommended, care must be taken not to use calcium ascorbate formulas, as this may lower magnesium levels (which is essential in all cases and types of premenstrual syndrome). PMS-E women usually tend to consume large amounts of dairy products. Animal fats should be avoided, as should any products containing yeast, because yeast has a stimulating effect on oestrogen activity. (*Science* 1984, Vol. 224, p. 109)

Excessive brain serotonin (5HT) can often cause aggressiveness, irritability and mood swings. Because oestrogen may already contribute to an elevation of those neurotransmitters, formulas containing tryptophan should be taken with care. While Vitamin B_3 (niacin or niacinamide) can be of some benefit, care must be taken against excesses in self prescribing. A certain amount of carbohydrates, about 30 g or the equivalent of one banana, tend to facilitate the transfer of tryptophan across the blood-brain barrier, as can any insulin-elevating food. But, of course, this is dependent on the amounts of tryptophan contained in the remaining portion of the meal. Foods containing high proportions of tryptophan should not be taken with sweets.

The liver helps to rid the body of excess oestrogen, so any food that decreases liver functions, such as hepatotoxic drugs, should be avoided or carefully monitored.

Insufficient amino acids (which provide the liver with fuel), B-complex deficiencies and anything but the most moderate intake of alcohol (1 or 2 drinks per day with meals) can aggravate PMS-E and all patients should be screened for a history of hepatitis and other liver diseases.

Vitamin B_{15} (pangamic acid) may be useful in such cases. Again, magnesium and Vitamin E, along with evening primrose oil are invaluable in this condition especially since Vitamin E (tocopherol) is said to produce some anti-oestrogenic effect.

Oestrogen can also affect the balance of renin (an enzyme which plays an important part in the maintenance of blood pressure) and angiotensin (a peptide which is capable of causing constriction of the blood vessels). Renin causes increased amounts of angiotensin to be produced which results in high blood pressure.

Foods high in Vitamin E

egg	peanuts
lettuce	salmon steak
margarine	sweet potato
mayonnaise	vegetables (dark green,
milk	leafy ones)
oils, cold-pressed	wheat germ
parsley	

Foods high in Vitamin B_{15} (pangamic acid)

almonds	rice bran
apricot kernels	rice shoots
liver	yeast (Brewer's)

ALLERGENS AND ADDICTIONS

The list of potential allergens is endless, but, apart from toxic chemicals, the most common offenders are corn, wheat, sugar, coffee, chocolate, milk, malt, barley and yeast.

If you look at the foods listed above carefully, you will notice that they are probably some of the most common ingredients that we use. We eat them very frequently, often without realising.

It is possible to become addicted to a substance because it is eaten too often or in large quantities. Most, if not all, of the common food allergies are 'masked' because they are, in fact, addictions.

As soon as the withdrawal symptoms start, one eats the offending food again and thereby successfully masks the allergy. Coffee addicts, chocaholics and cigarette smokers all feel better after ingesting their toxin. So beware, often the allergic food is one you actually like and eat a lot of.

---

3. PMS-A (allergy)

Almost the entire spectrum of symptoms may be caused by an underlying, undiagnosed or 'masked' allergy or intolerance to common foods or chemicals.

Hypersensitivities of this kind are often, but not always, mediated via the immune system and standard allergy profile tests are a good start in the diagnostic process involved. The standard tests should not be taken, however, as the complete answer unless a series of provocation-challenge tests follows.

The most common trigger foods and chemicals appear to be yeast, wheat, gluten, milk and house dust, although I have seen cases of PMS-A patients who were hypersensitive to their own lipstick (often an orris root allergy) or perfume or some common foods such as lettuce and potato.

4. PMS-C (candida)

Thrush (monilia), a common condition caused by a yeast fungus called Candida albicans, is responsible for a great many health problems. I have seen more women who suffer from premenstrual syndrome because of systemic candidiasis than almost any other single group.

These women should be treated for the underlying thrush first (avoid all alcohol and yeast-containing foods) and kept under observation for PMS symptoms. Only when, and if, the PMS symptoms do not disappear, should one begin to look for other possible causes for their menstrual problems.

5. PMS-H (hypoglycaemia)

These patients tend to suffer from wild fluctuations in blood-sugar levels. They are often very tired and feel dizzy and mentally confused, especially on awakening and mid-afternoon. Their symptoms tend to be worse when they do not eat and they are given to sugar binges.

Apart from a glucose-tolerance test, the most common symptoms and signs of this group are the timing and severity of their attacks in relation to the amount of food, especially sweets, that they eat. They can be prone to fainting spells and often cry for no apparent reason. They mimic classic 'neurotic' symptoms and are often called that by impatient husbands and doctors.

They are particularly sensitive to sugars and often have excessive insulin activity. Garlic, chromium and yeast supplements affect insulin activity and may aggravate this condition.

PMS-H sufferers are invariably deficient in magnesium and need strong supplements of Vitamin B and zinc. Zinc aids the synthesis and release of gamma linoleic acid (GLA) which reduces symptoms of PMS in general. Vitamin B_3 is used in the conversion of GLA into prostaglandin (PGE 1), which is a hormone-like substance that helps with both the physical and mental symptoms of premenstrual syndrome.

The oil of evening primrose is one of the best sources of linoleic acid and GLA (apart from breast milk) and this is probably one of the reasons why this supplement has proven so helpful in the treatment of premenstrual syndrome.

At the same time, animal fats antagonise some of these helpful processes and should, therefore, be avoided or drastically reduced, as should table salt.

Foods high in zinc

beef	mushrooms
bran	oatmeal
Brazil nuts	oysters
crab	pork
egg	pumpkin seeds
grains	rice, brown
herring	sunflower seeds
kidney	tuna
lamb	veal
milk	yeast (Brewer's)

Foods high in magnesium

almonds	Lima beans
apricots, dried	molasses
avocado	oatmeal
baked beans	peaches
barley	peanuts
beef	peas
Brazil nuts	pecans
carrots (raw)	pork
cashews	potato
chicken	rice
citrus fruits	sesame
corn	soya beans
crab	tomato (raw)
dates	vegetables
fish (flounder, salmon, tuna)	(dark green, leafy ones)
lentils	wheat germ

Some writers have suggested that ample amounts of unrefined grains and legumes can be helpful; however, our clinical experience has shown that this can sometimes be counter-productive. First of all, many patients have an intolerance to grains (especially bran, wheat and corn) and secondly, some of these products, such as the legumes, are particularly high in phytic acid which blocks the absorption of zinc. Zinc supplements taken on an empty stomach can help to circumvent this problem.

Each case is different because people could be intolerant to some foods and not others. An intolerance tends to irritate the gut walls and this will also cause problems with absorption.

Hypoglycaemics tend to fare better on a high protein diet but, at the same time, they should avoid excessive fats. Animal meats do contain antibiotics and oestrogen, and both these factors can aggravate hypoglycaemic sufferers.

One way to get around some of these problems is to include Spirulina in a dietary regimen that consists of small snacks with a good balance of vegetables and non-allergenic grains, such as brown rice and millet. Spirulina contains all the necessary amino acids without being derived from animal sources.

5. PMS-D *(depression)*

This group is characterised by severe premenstrual depression and, at times, suicidal tendencies. In most, if not all, cases one of the first practical things to do is to administer a Hoffer and Osmond diagnostic test to ascertain the possibility of suicide and to define quantitatively the role played by pure endogenous depression in the overall expression of psychological disturbance. It also helps to discover if the patient has an underlying psychiatric problem which is confused for, and often masked by, premenstrual syndrome.

Some of these patients may benefit from oral contraceptives as they tend to have a relatively high progesterone/oestrogen ratio. They are invariably deficient in or dependent on B-complex vitamins, especially Vitamin B_6, and magnesium.

Heavy-metal intoxication, especially lead, is common and many of these women find they are worse after physical exercise—especially jogging in a city. This is partly because they pass more polluted air through their lungs and partly because the decreased post-exertion pH of body fluids tends to leach out lead into the bloodstream.

Copper is also a problem because it may indirectly cause a lowering of some neurotransmitters in the brain.

PMS-D sufferers are probably the only premenstrual syndrome patients for whom we sometimes recommend tryptophan and when this is done we often add DL-phenylalanine and tyrosine to the supplement regimen.

They are usually badly affected by any forms of stress (the 'I can't cope' syndrome) but their adrenal involvement varies greatly. Many suffer from hypoadrenocorticism (adrenal exhaustion) and benefit from additional supplements of Vitamin B plus Siberian ginseng. A careful history check and some specialised tests can often single out this group.

Some, however, suffer from excessive adrenal stimulation, especially during the early phases of the syndrome, which in any case often precedes adrenal exhaustion. Vitamin B_5, ginseng and excessive Vitamin C may actually produce a temporary worsening of the symptoms when the adrenal glands are over-stimulated. One of the clues is that these patients are very cyclic in their responses to stress, which can vary from the need for total isolation and avoidance of sensory inputs (they don't even like to talk at the time) to the need for mental or physical stimulation.

7. PMS-F (fluid retention)

Although this group share many signs and symptoms with sufferers of PMS-E, the underlying hormonal-metabolic mechanism may be quite different.

Fluid retention, abdominal swelling, breast congestion, weight gain and cravings for salty and/or sweet foods are common to both groups. However, menstrual blood is less often clotty and tiredness is not a predominant feature.

Often excessive alcohol intake and decreased liver function exist along with a degree of hyperinsulinism in these patients. They are often under continuous although not necessarily excessive stress which, because it increases the secretion of aldosterone (a stress hormone which causes the body to retain sodium), will lead to further fluid retention.

It has been demonstrated that some PMS-F sufferers are deficient in dopamine (Kuchel D., Cuche J. L. *et al.*, 1977) which in turn may affect sodium and magnesium balance. For this reason tyrosine and DL-phenylalanine may prove useful.

Dietary guidelines

Almost all cases of premenstrual syndrome respond favourably to oil of evening primrose, magnesium, zinc, Vitamin E and Vitamin B_6 supplementation. In some cases, the vitamin ratios have to be altered. Fluid retention, for instance, does not appear to be influenced by oil of evening primrose while its response to Vitamin B_6 seems to be quite good.

Following are some basic dietary guidelines:

- People who produce excessive oestrogen and suffer from sub-clinical hypothyroidism may benefit from avoiding members of the cabbage family (Brussels sprouts, cauliflower, soya, peanuts) and animal meats, especially red meat.
- All sufferers from premenstrual syndrome should restrict high sugar foods, including honey, dried fruit, undiluted fruit juices and sweet desserts.
- Take plenty of Vitamin C, Vitamin B_6 and magnesium, and also a little zinc.
- Take a good Vitamin-B complex supplement but avoid those that contain too much folic acid (no more than 50 micrograms) and excessive PABA (no more than 50 milligrams).
- Alcohol, coffee, tea, chocolate and salt intake should be as low as possible.
- Be very wary of adopting a specific restrictive diet, especially if it varies greatly from your usual one. Before changing your diet, examine the possibility of food intolerances and allergies, because there is no point in being free of premenstrual syndrome if you end up with an irritable colon.

THE GOOD OIL—OIL OF EVENING PRIMROSE

When English physician Dr Caroline Shreeve ended up in the divorce court because her extreme irritability had made it impossible for her to get along with her husband, she decided to look at the reasons for her behaviour. For the previous five years she had suffered extreme symptoms of premenstrual syndrome.

Dr Shreeve decided it was time to look for a possible cure. She tried everything: fluid and salt restrictions—'helpful, but not enough'; yoga and relaxation—'wonderful at most times, but at that time many women don't feel like doing anything that sensible'; vitamin therapy—'certainly an integral part of any successful treatment but not sufficient for many people'; diuretics—'they can cause more trouble than they are worth'; progesterone—'very useful, but not all women who should respond to this treatment do so'; the pill—'too many worries about side effects'; tranquillisers—'they achieve nothing'; and Vitamin B_6—'useful only in those who are deficient in this vitamin to start with'. Dr Shreeve was getting nowhere fast.

In 1981 Dr Shreeve married again, this time a psychotherapist, and, during the same year, she attended an international medical symposium where she heard Dr Michael Brush of the St Thomas Hospital, London, talk about a series of double-blind, cross-over trials in the treatment of premenstrual syndrome with a flower!

To be more precise, it was with the extract of a bright yellow English flower called the evening primrose (*Oenothera biennis*). Its seeds are crushed and produce an oil which is a rich source of a rare essential fatty acid called gamma linoleic acid (GLA). (One of the few natural sources of GLA is breast milk.)

Essential fatty acids, or polyunsaturates, have the active ingredient linoleic acid from which the body makes GLA. However, as soon as a polyunsaturated oil is heated, deodorised, hydrogenated or otherwise artificially processed, the linoleic acid is changedinto a 'bad' form which actually blocks further synthesis of GLA.

In addition, diets high in animal fats and alcohol, insufficient in zinc, magnesium or Vitamin B_6, and viral infections and diabetes, can also block the synthesis of GLA.

(Cont.)

The Good Oil (Cont.)

GLA is converted into prostaglandin (PGE 1) which is a ubiquitous hormone-like substance that helps to reduce blood pressure, prevent inflammations, activate insulin, produce a sense of well-being in many people and relieve the physical and mental symptoms of premenstrual syndrome.

In fact, Dr Shreeve claims that a deficiency of GLA is one of the main causes of premenstrual syndrome and other symptoms associated with this syndrome. She also claims that the 'good oil' can reduce cholesterol levels, lower blood pressure, improve eczema, fix brittle nails, reduce the severity of hangovers, help in the treatment of hyperactivity and that it has been used experimentally in the treatment of multiple sclerosis.

Dr Shreeve has since written a book on premenstrual syndrome called *Premenstrual Syndrome, the Curse That Can Be Cured.*

8

HYPERACTIVITY AND CHILDREN'S LEARNING DIFFICULTIES

One of the difficult factors in understanding hyperactivity is distinguishing true hyperactive behaviour from the normal restlessness and curiosity of children.

While it is true that some of the symptoms of hyperactivity can be a normal extension of behaviour patterns, it is also clear that some children are being adversely affected by environmental and lifestyle factors. The difficulties experienced by these children, and their parents, make hyperactivity a distressing and serious problem, but one that can be cured.

Any form of abnormal behaviour, such as hyperactivity, can be the result of an enormous range of factors: emotional stress, difficult or restrictive environments, psychological or physical abuse. These and other psychodynamic possibilities should be properly evaluated by a competent professional, usually a child psychiatrist or psychologist. There is, however, a growing body of scientific evidence which shows that exposure to commonly-used chemicals (such as food additives), some nutrients and poor nutrition can cause allergies or intolerances in children.

Unfortunately, these allergies and intolerances not only cause behavioural problems but can also influence a child's ability to learn. Thus it is not uncommon to find that hyperactive children appear to be slow learners also. Paradoxically, this happens in spite of the fact that such children are usually very intelligent.

Difficult to believe? Just imagine you were trying to read and understand a legal paper or a scientific article while someone was tickling your ear or feet with a feather. The constant neurological distraction of the tickling would make it very difficult for you to concentrate and understand what you were reading irrespective of how intelligent you are! Allergies or intolerances to food, and sensitivities to chemicals act in the same way: they constantly irritate the nervous system of the child and make it difficult for them to concentrate and learn.

HYPERACTIVITY AND HEREDITY

Heredity cannot be ruled out as a factor contributing to hyperactivity. The boy-girl ratio for hyperactivity is 8:1 and it is thought by some psychiatrists that more boys suffer from food sensitivities because it is passed on to children via the mother's X chromosome (as with colour blindness and haemophilia), especially if it is a case of defective enzymes.

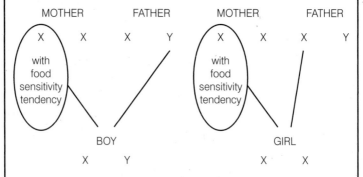

A boy has a 50 per cent chance of inheriting the X chromosome with food sensitivity and does not get an X chromosome from his father to mask this tendency.

The food sensitivity tendency inherited from the mother is recessive or masked by the father's non-defective X chromosome and therefore girls are unlikely to inherit this disorder. They may still, of course, suffer due to environmental factors rather than hereditary ones.

Signs and symptoms

Many hyperactive children tend to display some degree of anxiety or depression and are often tense. Sometimes these children are lethargic, tend to sleep or lie down doing nothing for hours, even days on end, only to emerge from their lethargy and start to behave very aggressively and destructively for no apparent reason.

Hyperactivity

Nervous system symptoms	**Other medical symptoms**
Hyperactive, wild, unrestrained, inattentive, disruptive	Stuffy or watery nose, sneezing, nose-rubbing,
Talkative	Aches in head, back, neck muscles; 'growing pains' or aches not related to exercise
Short attention span	Stomach problems, nausea, upset stomach, bad breath
Clumsiness, tremor, unco-ordination	Gassy stomach, belching
Restless legs, finger-tapping	Bloating, vomiting
Insomnia, nightmares, inability to fall asleep	Diarrhoea, constipation
Nervous, irritable, upset, short-tempered	Bladder problems, daytime or night-time, bed-wetting, urgency, burning or pain with urine
Highly strung, excitable, agitated	Pale or dark circles, or puffiness below eyes
Moody, tired, weak, exhausted, listless	Swollen glands or lymph nodes in neck
Depressed	Ear problems, repeated fluid behind eardrums, ringing ears
Easily moved to tears, easily hurt	Dizziness
Highly sensitive to odour, light, sound, pain, and/or cold	Excessive perspiration, low grade fever

(Cont.)

Hyperactivity (Cont.)

Behavioural signs and symptoms
Crib rocking and head knocking during infancy
Aggressive and/or disruptive at home and school
Touches everything and everybody
Disturbs other children
Does not respond to discipline
Unpredictable behaviour
Panics easily, throws tantrums
Whatever he or she wants, it is NOW!
Fidgets
Can't sit still
Does not finish projects
Wears out furniture, toys, etc. Destructive.
Fights with other children
Refuses to follow directions
Clumsy—has difficulties with such things as doing up buttons or
   tying up shoelaces
Usually very intelligent but has difficulties learning
Hard to put to bed and sleep
Wakes up early
Lies
Bed wets
Sometimes has speech difficulties

Some children are quite allergic and suffer from runny noses, throat mucus, sinusitis, hay fever, asthma, skin rashes and digestive problems such as loose bowels, diarrhoea or constipation. They often display abdominal bloating after eating and their eyes tend to be watery and sometimes red and sore, especially on awakening.

Not every hyperactive child exhibits all, or even the majority, of these symptoms. But if enough of them are present there is a possibility that your child suffers from hyperactivity.

Causes

Sensitivity to food additives

Probably the best known scientist involved in research on the causes of hyperactivity was Dr Ben Feingold of the Kaiser Permanent Medical Center in San Francisco, California. In the 1960s Dr Feingold discovered that some chemicals added to our food could provoke a reaction in susceptible children which manifests itself in hyperactive behaviour.

RED FOOD COLOURING

While working on the problem of irritation caused by flea bites, Dr Feingold found that colourings, especially red ones, were a major factor in hyperactive behaviour. This is not as bizarre as it sounds, because cochineal, the traditional red cake colouring, is, or was, made from the crushed bodies of tiny cactus-eating insects. It is the secretions made in the flea's body that cause most of the irritation when one is bitten.

Dr Feingold claimed he had irrefutably proved a cause-and-effect relationship between food additives and hyperactive behaviour. The most convincing proof was the ability to switch off and then provoke the reaction in hyperactive children by withholding and later re-administering the offending substance.

Millions of children all over the world have gone on the 'Feingold diet' and benefited from it. Dr Feingold also discovered that many children are unusually sensitive to a chemical 'cousin' of salicylate (the common ingredient in aspirin), which is found in some fruits and vegetables.

Feingold's recommended diet consisted of eliminating all foods that are coloured, preserved, tinned, instant, or are known to contain chemical additives. At the same time, all foods containing the natural salicylates are also avoided. These include almonds, apples, apricots, blackberries, cloves, cucumbers, pickles, currants, gooseberries, raisins, mint flavours, nectarines, oranges, peaches, plums, prunes, raspberries, strawberries, teas of any kind, tomatoes and oil of wintergreen.

The Feingold diet is responsible for curing up to about 40 per cent of hyperactive children and as many as 60 per cent can be helped. However, it is also a fact that many children fail to respond, or respond only partially, to this regimen.

What, then, is the reason for this failure rate? At the time of Dr Feingold's research, other scientists were busy looking into the role played by nutrients, smells, fumes, heavy metals and other substances in altering human behaviour. Several scientists in centres in the United States, Europe and Australia were becoming aware of a greater range of possible factors.

Hypoglycaemia

It was also found that a large number of hyperactive children suffer from abnormal fluctuations in their blood-sugar levels: they were hypoglycaemic.

Hypoglycaemia means 'low blood sugar' and results when sugars, refined carbohydrates or other blood-sugar elevating substances are eaten (especially on an empty stomach). The body overreacts by producing chemicals that send blood-sugar levels plummeting. For a number of reasons the blood sugar may fail to return to normal levels unless further amounts of sweets are eaten. During this period, while levels are low, the individual is in a state of biochemical stress. Very much like a drug addict or alcoholic, they need another shot. Often these people are classified as 'sugarholics'— they are addicted to substances which elevate their blood sugar.

All these metabolic ups and downs unsettle the nervous system and can cause a variety of behavioural symptoms, including hyperactivity. They often make it impossible for the child to concentrate or study and he quickly falls behind in his school work.

It is also important to understand that, in some individuals, the blood-sugar levels may drop from a high level to reasonably normal limits, but they drop so fast that the nervous system is adversely affected. Also one must consider that what is a normal level for one individual may be too low for another.

The other essential point is that although sugar may trigger the drop, any substance to which the individual is sensitive (allergic or intolerant) may cause the blood-sugar levels to fall. Sometimes, people suffering from this problem show the opposite symptoms to hyperactivity. They are always tired, sleepy and lethargic, and never get anything done.

DOUBLE-BLIND TESTS

By 1950, Dr William Crook, another leading figure in environmental allergies, was performing the first of the 'double-blind' studies in this area, with a young patient who had a problem with milk.

In a double-blind test nobody—patient, parents or doctor— knows which medication is a placebo (a harmless substance given deliberately) and which is the suspect substance.

In this case, Dr Crook's patient felt quite well for the first two weeks, but after the change to the second lot of tablets in week three (these were the ones containing milk), symptoms such as stuffy nose, fatigue, stomach aches, headaches, depression and irritability reappeared within three days.

Sensitivities to moulds, fungi, ferments and yeasts

It was then found that quite a few hyperactive children were also hypersensitive or allergic to fungi. After they were placed on a yeast or mould-free diet, given antifungals when needed, and their environment was cleared of mould, the children were tested and desensitised. Only then did their behaviour improve.

Mineral deficiencies or imbalances

This can be caused by excessive ingestion of or contamination by minerals.

Excessive copper can come from the drinking water (via copper piping) or from food (via copper saucepans) leading to a relative deficiency of zinc (because zinc competes with copper for absorption). Copper generally tends to increase nervous excitation, whereas zinc has a calming effect on nerves. Frozen vegetables are usually deficient in zinc, and vegetarian diets that have too much soya beans can boost copper to unacceptable levels.

Heavy metal intoxication

There are some people so sensitive to certain fumes and odours that it causes them to behave strangely. I can recall one case where a child was affected by his father's aftershave lotion.

JUNK FOOD AND HYPOGLYCAEMIA

In a series of tests at a school for problem children in the western suburbs of Sydney—an area renowned for high levels of air pollution, children with allergies, asthma and learning difficulties—more than 75 per cent of children tested were found to be hypoglycaemic.

When these fluctuations were levelled out by eliminating junk foods and sugars from the diet and including Vitamin C, Vitamin B, magnesium and zinc, most of the children improved remarkably. Another series of investigations found these children to be equally sensitive to fructose (the sugar commonly found in fruits) and to sucrose (cane sugar). A small number were found to react badly to dried fruits.

A diet eliminating all sugars, including honey and dried fruits, helped a considerable number of hyperactive children. Meanwhile, quite coincidentally, another suspect substance was uncovered—yeast.

More common sources of irritation can be gas stoves, aerosol sprays and perfumes and, of course, lead from exhaust fumes. Is your child's playground by a busy main road or, worse still, at an intersection? Do you buy fruit and vegetables from street-corner barrows? If so, these may be sources of unwanted heavy metals.

Sensitivity to inhaled chemicals

Deodorant sprays, hairsprays, oven-cleaners and dozens of commonly used household products and substances found in your child's school may be causing an allergic reaction and therefore hyperactive symptoms.

Treatment

Many hyperactive children may be able to eat some or all of the fruits and vegetables excluded by the Feingold diet after they have eliminated some of the other contributing factors discussed under 'Causes' in the previous pages.

It seems that so many allergies or intolerances happen because of a combination of factors. If a child is allergic to mould, dust or pollens, the sensitivity to salicylates may be reduced dramatically after these other allergies have been taken care of. The opposite is also true. A child who continues to eat something that he or she is allergic to is more likely to exhibit symptoms when he or she is exposed to pollens or other air-borne factors.

Once placed on the appropriate diet, many of those allergic children can tolerate some exposure to dust, pollens and other substances without being severely affected. In many cases, when a sensitivity has been established, it is possible that the child will lose it after several months. This is more common with foods or inhalant allergies than with chemical food additives.

It is sometimes possible to desensitise sufferers with allergy drops under the tongue, whereas at other times a neutralisation technique known as serial titration is called for.

Serial titration is carried out by provoking the symptoms with an extract of the suspect substance and then progressively diluting the extract. Each dilution is given to the patient to ascertain if it can switch off or neutralise the symptoms. If it fails to do so, it is further diluted until a dilution of the extract is found that is capable of stopping the symptom. A vaccine is then prepared and this is taken by the patient to neutralise the allergy.

After a suitable time, some of these children are able to start eating the offending foods on a four-day rotation diet; that is, the food can be eaten once in every four days.

I want to make it very clear that all I have said so far must not be taken to mean that it is a case of 'either-or'. It is not uncommon that a hyperactive child is either hypoglycaemic or sensitive to chemicals, or suffers from gluten sensitivity, or is allergic to environmental factors. Each of these can be a cause, or be just one factor in the whole problem.

It can often happen that an individual has several sensitivities or allergies and that the one problem has several causes. In some cases every one of them has to be eliminated before the child will function normally again. In other cases, taking care of the major ones will sufficiently enhance the body's own ability to overcome the remaining sensitivities to a point where they do not cause any symptoms.

Above all, a thorough evaluation is mandatory for each case. Remember, every one of us is a unique individual, biochemically as well as psychologically.

The Feingold diet

After you have removed all foods with artificial colourings and flavourings from your child's diet, as Dr Feingold recommends on page 141, the next step is to check on common, everyday foods as these may be involved in a masked intolerance.

Skin allergy tests are not very helpful in identifying food sensitivities although they are useful in detecting allergies to pollen, house dust, mites, animal dander and other inhaled substances. Intradermal and sublingual tests, however, are much more likely to indicate food sensitivities with the added advantage that the therapist is then able to prepare desensitising vaccines (drops) or other neutralising therapy.

Milk, as most parents have heard, is a very popular suspect allergen, and it is closely followed by grains, especially gluten-containing ones like wheat, rye, oats and malt. Other foods such as sugar, peas, beans, citrus fruits, beef, pork, chicken and potato may also be problems. By eliminating all these foods one at a time, you may find that your child's symptoms improve by the fourth or fifth day; but, if not, persevere for up to three weeks.

To find out exactly which food or foods have been causing problems, introduce them one at a time to see whether the symptoms return. There are tests that can be done by trained practitioners, but they are fairly controversial in the eyes of orthodox physicians. They include the now very old and unreliable cytotoxic test, the RAST test, the pulse test and the kinesiology test.

MASKED INTOLERANCES—WHAT ARE THEY?

An intolerance or allergy can be masked by continual intake of the allergenic substance. If you are addicted to anything, every time you take another dose you'll feel better because you avoid the withdrawal symptoms.

The addiction 'masks' the reality that the substance is toxic to you. In the same way, eating something to which you are allergic several times each day will tend to 'mask' the symptoms of the allergic reaction. This does not apply to everyone who is allergic but, if it does, the individual will not be aware that he or she is allergic.

Oligo-antigenic diet

A simple way to determine whether your child is suffering a food allergy is to adopt a strict elimination diet called an Oligo-antigenic diet.

Place the child on basic multi-vitamin and mineral supplements plus a little zinc and magnesium. Then continue with a strict diet that excludes potentially allergenic foods. The basis of the diet includes food such as sweet potatoes, cabbage, carrots, free range lamb or turkey, pears and purified water. After a few weeks you should be able to notice the change in the child's behaviour.

Once you've established that the child is better, start to reintroduce foods—one per day. Leave wheat grain products, yeast and sugar until last. If any food is responsible or even a contributing factor, you will know by the change in the child's behaviour. This is one way you can establish which are safe foods and which are not.

Preventative measures

One way to lessen the possibility of your child acquiring a food allergy or intolerance is to practise preventative medicine and take precautions during pregnancy.

The following steps will help you to establish the best possible environment for your child during pregnancy and childhood.

During pregnancy

It is very important to eat a well-balanced diet. Vary your diet and avoid eating large quantities of any single food, especially those you dislike or those which disagree with you.

There is some evidence from Sweden that if you are sensitive to milk then it will probably upset your baby as well. Calcium is needed during pregnancy and if you cannot drink milk, it is available in yoghurt, some vegetables and certain hard cheeses.

If you find that you are craving a certain type of food, it is usually an indication that your diet is deficient in a vitamin or mineral found in that food. It is necessary to take a good hard look at what you are eating and it may be advisable to consider vitamin and mineral supplements.

Remember also that vegetables will lose fewer vitamins and minerals when they are put through the juice extractor rather than being overcooked.

A varied diet also helps build up digestive enzymes for passing on to your baby through your breast milk.

After your child is born

It is very important to breast-feed. Try to arrange for your baby to be put onto your breast as soon as possible after the birth so that they benefit from the colostrum, the thickish yellow substance that comes from the nipples just before the milk starts flowing. Colostrum plays a very important part in helping to build up protective bacteria in the baby's digestive tract and it also gives some immune protection.

Don't begin feeding your baby on solids too soon. Cereal is liable to be a major hazard, since it generally contains wheat and most canned baby dinners contain wheat flour as a thickener. There has, however, been a healthy move towards reducing sugar, salt and monosodium glutamate in most baby food products. If you suspect your baby may be prone to food allergies or sensitivities, avoid chocolate and egg until the baby is nine months or older.

If weaning to cows' milk or cows' milk formulae causes diarrhoea or any other adverse symptoms, remove it from the baby's diet completely until the symptoms subside. This also goes for junkets, yoghurt, puddings and probably even cheese. If your baby has difficulty with cows' milk and you are not breast-feeding, vegetable juices such as carrot juice, nut and seed milks, and goats' milk are good alternative sources of calcium.

It is very important to give your baby a wide variety of natural foods and to avoid processed or canned foods. Rotate and diversify your baby's diet as much as possible because a food allergy or intolerance is much more likely to develop if a food is taken every day.

It is true that babies are initially wary of new foods. However, you can't mistake real, determined dislike and no matter how wholesome a food is, do not persevere with it if it is causing distress. This is how hidden or masked allergies start.

9

NEUROTOXINS—POLLUTION, CHEMICALS AND YOUR BRAIN

The diagnosis of human illness is, in many ways, an exercise in the detection of biochemical, psychological or physiological disturbances in an individual. People only become aware of the effects of such disturbances when symptoms of this disturbance become apparent. Symptoms are the body's own warning signals that tell us something is amiss.

We become ill for many different reasons: stress, trauma, malignant cells, infectious agents (viruses, bacteria, fungi, etc.) or simply because we do not receive sufficient nutrients to enable our body to ward off an attack. Whatever the causes, symptoms can vary greatly from person to person and from illness to illness. Of course, the symptoms one actually 'feels' can have their origin in different parts of the body.

We tend to think of body functions only in terms of the organs responsible for them. Because of the particular orientation of orthodox medical education, physicians often think of organ functions as if each were a separate entity. We talk about heart functions, kidney functions and lung functions, almost as if these organs existed as independent, self-contained units. But, in fact, each organ is totally dependent on every other organ. For example, it is pointless to talk about heart disease as if the heart existed in total isolation: the heart's blood supply depends on healthy circulation and blood is useless unless it is full of the necessary ingredients for life—nutrients from the foods we eat, the gases we breathe and the fluids we drink. To some extent, our circulation is also dependent on physical activity which can be affected by anything from our sex life to our working conditions.

Brain functions are largely regulated by the hormones the brain produces from amino acids present in the food we eat and the brain cannot get these unless the foods are digested and absorbed. However, the brain is a very delicate organ and its intricate hormonal system can become unbalanced; its synchronicity can be thrown out of kilter; and its regulatory neurotransmitter chemicals can be antagonised, deactivated or inhibited by a considerable number of substances—natural or otherwise.

There is a particular class of chemicals called neurotoxins which can damage the nervous system and can, therefore, cause almost any emotional or 'behavioural' symptom—from hallucinations to depression, from sleeplessness to dementia and from memory loss to psychosis.

Changes brought about by neurotoxins are so subtle and treacherous that most people who are affected by them have no idea what is causing their symptoms. Often their doctors are equally unaware of the real cause of the problem and they begin to search for physical causes for each of the symptoms that might, in fact, be the early warnings of neurotoxicity.

Tingling and numbness of the fingers or toes, slight tremors or a 'shaky' feeling, slight unco-ordination, impotence, and decreased sensations of touch, are all characteristics of neurotoxicity. Later, perhaps years after the initial exposure to a neurotoxin, there may be some general pains, problems with vision, a decreased sense of smell and taste, lowered alertness, loss of memory, lethargy, irritability and even depression, hallucinations or psychosis—or a combination of any of these.

In some cases, a few of these effects are irreversible because of the difficulties of repairing or replacing damaged or lost cells. The consequences on the human brain are therefore almost invariably permanent. Because the nature of the presenting symptoms are so diverse, these are often attributed to an excessive workload, advancing age or even stress. Let us now take a look at some of the neurotoxins in our environment.

POLLUTION AND LEARNING DIFFICULTIES IN CHILDREN

Children are particularly susceptible to toxins of all kinds. Because learning is such an essential part of growing up, the effects of pollution on brain functions can be devastating in a child.

Usually the first signs are what we would normally call altered behaviour, but behaviour is such an individualistic phenomenon that few parents (or even teachers) are aware of the problem until it is too late.

The Select Committee on Nutrition and Human Needs of the United States Senate 95th Congress stated:

The early symptoms of lead poisoning are subtle, subjective and non-specific and therefore not so easily recognised in children. In children such mild symptoms are often either overlooked or attributed to other diseased states, so that poisoning due to lead is more likely to be recognised first at a late or severe stage on the basis of nervous system involvement.

In other words, by the time we are aware that our children are suffering from subtle pollutants it may be too late.

Ethoxyethanol

This is a widely used industrial solvent related to the alcohol found in lacquers, dyes, varnish removers and many other industrial processes. It has always been regarded as 'safe' and, indeed, when the compound was extensively tested in laboratory animals, it was shown to produce no toxic effects. Even pregnant rats did not suffer when exposed to doses equivalent to half the allowable limits. But their offspring did! Subsequent tests showed significant changes in brain chemistry and after-birth behaviour.

The implications of the following experiment are also interesting. B. K. Nelson, a scientist at the National Institute for Occupational Safety and Health in America, gave a group of pregnant rats the same amount of ethoxyethanol which had been shown to be safe for them but toxic to their offspring. At the same time he mixed a little alcohol into their drinking water. He discovered that the effects of this combination on the brain neurochemistry of their offspring were twice as severe as those caused by ethoxyethanol alone.

There are rather frightening implications because of this phenomenon. It is quite possible that a great many people who are infrequently exposed to small amounts of ethoxyethanol may suffer no symptoms—at least no observable ones—from such exposure. However, if the same people consume regular amounts of alcohol in addition to being exposed to ethoxyethanol, although they are not directly harmed, the toxicity of ethoxyethanol is such that their children may suffer serious neurological consequences.

Carbon disulphide

Discovered in the latter part of the 18th century, carbon disulphide (CS_2) was originally used as a general anaesthetic. J. Simpson, a Scottish surgeon, reported in 1840 that he was no longer using it because it caused hallucinations, headaches and nausea in his patients. Within a few years CS_2 was used extensively as a solvent in industrial processes. It was then discovered that CS_2 could 'soften' rubber at any temperature, thus making it possible to manufacture many things such as raincoats, rubber toys and balloons. Of course, anyone working with this substance was exposed to its deadly fumes.

Already by 1856 the writings of the Frenchman Dr Auguste Delpeech contained a warning:

> He who works in the 'sulphur' is no longer a man. He may still make a living from day to day in unskilled labour. He will never be able to establish an independent position for himself. The depressing influence of the carbon sulphide upon his will-power, the painful consequences of his indifference, and the loss of his memory, prevent him from entering another occupation.

The doctor also described how some of the workers' children, who spent a few days playing near their fathers while they worked, were 'stricken with a type of raging delirium'.

Alan Anderson, writing in *Psychology Today*, tells us that in 1902 a British publication, *Dangerous Trades*, described a factory in which the windows were barred to prevent crazed workers from leaping forth during their frequent delirious attacks!

Meanwhile the rubber industry has developed causing untold thousands of unsuspecting workers to lose their health and sanity.

In Finland, workers in modern, well-ventilated and clean rayon factories have been tested and shown to have lost some neuromuscular speed, intelligence and psychomotor ability.

Nitrates

Although nitrates themselves are not particularly toxic, when they change to nitrites or nitrosamines they can become quite dangerous. They are suspected of being carcinogenic. However, a lesser known and just as frightening capacity of nitrites is that of causing methaemoglobinaemia—a condition in which blood no longer carries an adequate amount of oxygen. A small child affected with this disease may turn blue and suffer permanent brain damage as a result. As the child grows up, the impairment may show in several ways. Nitrates thus become neurotoxic.

Feeding babies with formulas made up with well water is not recommended as these may have a high content of nitrates. Well water can easily become contaminated by pesticides and other chemicals which are used in agriculture. Sometimes animal wastes can be high in nitrate content and this may affect local water supplies. Methaemoglobinaemia can also be caused by air that has been polluted by vanadium.

Volatile fuels

According to some studies, workers exposed to jet fuels have poor scores in behavioural tests that demand a high degree of concentration. Statistically, such workers were found to have more psychiatric illnesses and symptoms of depression and neurotic behaviour.

Similar results were obtained in studies of people exposed to paint solvents. A Scandinavian study reported in *Psychology Today* (July, 1982) revealed that when fifty-two house painters were studied they scored lower than control on tests of intellectual capacity, psychomotor co-ordination, memory and reaction time. Totally oblivious of the danger, the workers sometimes washed their hands in methyl-n-butyl ketone, a powerful neurotoxin capable of severely damaging the central nervous system.

Surgeons and other operating theatre personnel are often exposed to anaesthetic gases which can escape from pressure-relief valves used during operations. Nitrous oxide and halothane, two anaesthetic gases, when inhaled in concentrations as low as fifty parts per million and one part per million respectively, can affect short-term memory, visual perception, acuity and cognitive motor responses—the very skills needed in an operating theatre!

Mercury

Mercury, or quicksilver, has always been regarded as somewhat magical because of its unique property—it is the only metal to be liquid at room temperature.

Its toxic properties have been well known since medieval times and it has been used extensively as a poison. It has been said that Napoleon, Ivan the Terrible and Charles II of England all died of mercury poisoning. Records exist to show that in the year 1700 a citizen of Finale, a small town in Italy, sought an injunction against a factory making mercury chloride because its fumes were killing the inhabitants.

A diagnosis of mercury poisoning is difficult to make. One of the problems is that damage may happen before the symptoms manifest; however, it is not apparent until neurological damage has already occurred. So, unfortunately, the accepted daily intake or exposure is that which is enough to cause symptoms.

An article in *Science* (1982, Vol. 177, p. 621) reported that, because foetal tissue is particularly susceptible to damage by chemicals and heavy metals, large doses of mercury were given to pregnant mice to test toxicity. All litters tested were born apparently healthy, they developed well and there appeared to be no difference between the mercury-injected mice and the untreated ones.

Indeed, when the respective brain sizes and neurotransmitter enzyme content were measured two months after birth, everything appeared quite normal. However, when these animals underwent subsequent behavioural tests, the researchers were in for a rude shock. Mice that had been given the mercury showed aberrant behaviour patterns.

Instead of exploring a new piece of territory like the control animals, they sat around listlessly and showed no interest whatsoever in their surroundings. When some of them did eventually start to move around they often walked backwards! The affected animals also showed a greatly reduced desire to groom themselves. The researchers then put the mice through normal swimming tests. Untreated mice learned to swim while the mercury-exposed mice swam poorly and periodically lapsed into bouts of neuromuscular unco-ordination.

Strangely enough, mercury was probably the first metal compound to be employed therapeutically and Hippocrates is believed to have prescribed mercury sulphide as a medication. During the 16th century it was extensively used to treat syphilis and someone with a sense of humour noted that 'a night with Venus might lead to a lifetime with mercury'.

Known as a toxic time bomb, dental fillings (which can be made from mercury) can slowly but insidiously poison an individual to the point where his or her immune system is working well below normal. The effects can be wide ranging and lead to all sorts of diseases.

HEAVY METALS AND THEIR EFFECTS

Arsenic	giddiness, headaches, general weakness, fatigue
Boron	restlessness, unco-ordination, aggressiveness, jitteriness and disorientation
Cadmium	fatigue, lack of taste and smell dysfunctions, increased heart disease risk

(Cont.)

Heavy Metals and Their Effects (Cont.)

Copper	irritability, poor concentration, hyperactivity
Manganese	psychiatric symptoms (French miners exposed to manganese showed symptoms indistinguishable from schizophrenia)
Mercury	tremors, unco-ordination, speech problems, psychiatric problems
Nickel	headaches, insomnia, delirium, irritability
Selenium	dizziness, lassitude, depression, fatigue
Tin	limb weakness, vertigo, photophobia
Pesticides in general	neurological, metabolic and psychiatric disturbances
Chlorine	skin rashes, lethargy, allergic reactions
Nitrates	possibly carcinogenic

Mercury and vegetarian diet

The people most at risk from the effect of mercury poisoning are strict vegetarians or vegans because mercury combines with sulphur-containing proteins.

The principal sources of methionine, one of the main sulphur amino acids, are eggs, meats, fish, poultry and dairy foods. Diets high in methionine, and other sulphur amino acids which are often made from methionine, afford some protection against mercury poisoning. However, this type of diet places a great strain on the body's reserves of Vitamin B_6 (pyridoxine) and this should always be taken as a supplement.

Mercury also affects the body's levels of Vitamin C, by reducing its level within the brain. One of the therapeutic uses of Vitamin C in treating heavy metal intoxication is the ability for this vitamin to form complexes with metals which are then taken out of the body via the urinary system.

Foods high in Vitamin B$_6$ (pyridoxine)

avocado

barley

beans

Brazil nuts

carrot

cheese

cow's milk

crab

egg

fish (cod, halibut,
    herring, mackerel,
    salmon, sardines, tuna)

lentils

Lima beans

liver (pork)

meat (beef, ham, pork)

milk

molasses

oranges

peanuts

peas

potato

prunes

rice

soya bean

spinach

sunflower seeds

wheat bran

wheat germ

wholemeal flour

yeast (Brewer's)

Foods high in Vitamin C (ascorbic acid)

alfalfa

banana

berries (blueberries,
    gooseberries, raspberries
    and strawberries)

Brazil nuts

broccoli

brussels sprouts

cabbage

cantaloupe melon

capsicum

cauliflower

citrus fruit (lemons,
    oranges, tomatoes)

guava

kidney

liver (beef)

oysters

potato

spinach

sweet potato

vegetables
    (green leafy ones)

watermelon

Selenium

Selenium combines with mercury, so a diet or intake of water containing adequate selenium gives some protection.

Selenium itself can be highly poisonous so dietary supplements are not recommended in large doses unless under supervision. Selenium is, nevertheless, a very important and essential mineral. People who drink water with low selenium content or who otherwise acquire selenium deficiency have been found to be prone to cardiovascular disease. Several reports have also linked cancer with a selenium-deficient diet but an excess intake is just as bad and, in this case, far worse than taking in too little.

We know that selenium can pollute water in areas where selenium-rich soil is irrigated. When animals eat the plants that grow there, the metal damages the foetus and, as with thalidomide, can cause the birth of deformed offspring. Sulphur supplements do not necessarily provide a shield against the mercury-induced catastrophe because an effective antidote must provide the body with a sulphur-containing protein, not inorganic sulphur.

IS SELENIUM AN ESSENTIAL MINERAL OR A TOXIC METAL?

An editorial article by David Rutolo which appeared in the *International Clinical Nutrition Review* in July 1983 asked: 'Is selenium an essential mineral or a toxic metal?'

The article reported on a heart condition called 'Keshan disease' which caused a large number of deaths in China during the 1970s. Researchers discovered that a major contributing factor to this rare condition was a lack of selenium in the diet and, after a vigorous programme of corrective supplements, the disease was practically wiped out.

This, however, is only one half of the story. There was also another incident some 20 years before when a group of inhabitants from five Chinese villages were affected by an endemic disease of unknown origin. This disease caused loss of hair and nails and neurological

(Cont.)

Is Selenium an Essential Mineral (Cont.)

impairments. When the inhabitants of these villages were moved to another area the physical symptoms disappeared. Those with neurological symptoms needed a longer time to recover.

At first a corn fungus was suspected, however selenium toxicity was later demonstrated to be the cause of the disease. Apparently, the outbreak of toxicity followed a drought which caused the failure of a rice crop, thereby forcing the villagers to eat more vegetables and maize which were high in selenium, and fewer protein foods. (*American Journal of Clinical Nutrition*)

Selenium levels in the hair, blood and urine reflect the selenium status of the population. The villagers with selenium toxicity had hair selenium levels one hundred times higher than usual and four hundred times higher than the people in the selenium-deficient areas where the Keshan disease occurred.

Pesticides

Pesticides encompass a great number of different agents including insecticides, fungicides, fumigants and rodenticides.

The first pesticide to be commonly used was not the invention of some perverse chemist but one of the ancient Chinese. Called pyrethrum, it was brought to Europe from China by Marco Polo in the 13th century. Although a natural compound, pyrethrum is a powerful allergen and a large number of people are unable to tolerate it. Asthmatics and those suffering from sinusitis seem to be the most easily affected, although I have seen many hyperactive children who would appear to be hypersensitive to it.

Probably the most famous, or infamous, pesticide of all is DDT—a chlorinated hydrocarbon which is toxic to the nervous system and does not decompose easily. It can be stored in living tissues for a very long time and in many parts of the world investigators have found that breast-feeding mothers sometimes inadvertently transmit enormous amounts of pesticides to their infants.

According to a 1999 report by the World Wildlife Fund, the breast milk of women in the UK has been found to contain up to forty times more pesticides than the maximum levels allowed for cows' milk by the World Health Organisation.

DDT interferes with calcium absorption and this can result in thin skulls, weak bones, muscular spasms and mental retardation. DDT is no longer used in developed countries, but is still in use in various parts of the developing world. However, the pesticides that replaced DDT turned out to be even more dangerous. Organophosphates are a type of insecticide or pesticide specifically toxic for the nerves because they affect acetylcholine, which is the main agent for nerve transmission to muscles. A study set up by the World Health Organisation has shown that a diet deficient in acetylcholine will increase a person's susceptibility to the dangers of pesticides. One pesticide in particular, Captan, is almost harmless to a well-nourished person but becomes deadly to someone with a protein-deficient diet.

The type of protein in the diet is also important. Animals raised on soya proteins tend to be deficient in methionine and have a high copper-to-zinc ratio. Such animals are not well protected against mercury poisoning because most anti-chemical activities in the body need sulphur-containing proteins. If the soya beans have been sprayed with any pesticides, as is often the case, the situation can be quite dangerous.

PESTICIDE LEVELS IN OUR BODIES

It now seems certain that every new baby born in Australia comes into the world with clearly discernible levels of pesticide in its body, according to a scientific analysis by the director of Maternal and Child Health in Queensland, Dr Jean McFarlane. In a 1978 survey of 170 mothers in and around Brisbane, 100%, that is every one of them, was found to have pesticides in their milk. When the children were tested by Dr McFarlane, again the result was 100%. There is enough going to support the view that all Australians have pesticides in their bodies; you, me—everybody—the whole community at large, even babies.

H. Lunn, *The Australian*, 18 January 1980

Soya is also marginally deficient in chromium, another factor that may contribute to ill-health if your diet relies heavily on that food. A chromium deficiency affects the body's capacity to make insulin and this can destabilise the blood sugar regulating mechanisms of the body. Rats raised on soya proteins tend to grow poorly and lose their liver reserves of Vitamin A when exposed to pesticides.

Some countries, particularly the USA and Sweden, have now acted to ban and phase out many of these dangerous pesticides. Alternatives have been developed but there are doubts about the effectiveness of some, and others may prove to be as toxic as their predecessors.

The fibre factor

Although the consumption of high-fibre foods is generally recommended and is normally beneficial to health, it must also be remembered that excessive fibre can cause some proteins to be malabsorbed. If this happens while a person is on a low-protein diet, exposure to pesticides can be fatal. This is an important factor that should be borne in mind when a vegetarian buys a farm for his own use.

Another point worth remembering, especially by those naturopaths who practise extensive fasting therapy, is that most pesticides, especially chlorinated hydrocarbons, accumulate in body fats. During prolonged fasting, these fat stores are broken down for energy, and pesticides, especially DDT, can infiltrate the blood, producing concentrations high enough to become dangerous.

Manganese

This is another potentially toxic metal. It is added to jet fuel to make the outpouring smoke less black—reducing the size of airborne particles so that they tend to disperse without being quite so visible. The particles, however, can penetrate lung tissue and cause serious respiratory and neurological damage.

Manganese is also used in ordinary petrol as a replacement for lead but it is doubtful if this is of any health advantage. For example, people employed in the manufacture of dry cell batteries are said to be at risk of developing paralysis as a result of exposure to manganese.

A brochure distributed by a leading hair analysis centre in the United States described the symptoms of manganese toxicity as very similar to, if not indistinguishable from, those of schizophrenia but adds that 'symptomatic deficiency of manganese has not been demonstrated in humans'.

Paradoxically, the use of manganese is invaluable in counteracting some of the side effects of phenothiazines, a group of psychiatric drugs that produce a syndrome called tardive dyskinesia. When used together with other vitamins, notably niacin, manganese is said to treat this disease quite successfully.

All in all, manganese seems to be a potentially toxic substance that can, nevertheless, be used effectively in the treatment of several diseases. It has been used extensively in orthomolecular psychiatry but, as I have pointed out, its widespread use as a supplement in high doses is potentially dangerous.

Trichloroethane

This rather frightening-sounding chemical may seem remote but is, in fact, a common thinner used in products such as Liquid Paper. It is one of the milder chlorinated hydrocarbons which acts as a thinner by keeping particles light and easily spreadable.

Hydrocarbons and fluorocarbons can, if inhaled in large enough quantities, cause symptoms similar to those which follow alcohol intoxication. They also cause headaches, ringing in the ears and hallucinations—not unlike those triggered by LSD. If enough hydrocarbons are inhaled, convulsions and eventually a state of coma may be the unhappy result.

Many people are unwittingly exposed to hydrocarbon and fluorocarbon fumes. Sensitive individuals, especially children, can suffer from twitching muscles and hyperactive reflexes as a result. Those who are hypersensitive or allergic to these compounds may also suffer extreme behavioural disorders because of exposure.

Lighter fluid, correction fluids, fly sprays, paint strippers and even cough medicines and car sickness pills contain hydrocarbons and fluorocarbons. They can be, and often are, abused by young people seeking a 'high'.

Toxins and the environment

Traditional definitions of toxicology for the most part encompass damage to the various body tissues and the likelihood of death. However, in the past few decades we have seen the focus shifting to environmental issues and concern with the consequences of long-term exposure to low levels of chemicals. Many scientific investigators, including myself, feel that one of the main criteria in investigating toxicity is that of 'functions'.

Since function defines life, and since many toxic substances disrupt functions, the effects of exposure should be studied by examining changes in various functions brought about by exposure. Behavioural toxicology is in fact a measurement of subtle functional disorders.

Within this frame of reference, lead poisoning can be seen as a major hazard to behavioural and mental health. A report on lead by the American National Research Council describes the medical and biological effects of environmental pollutants (Select Committee on Nutrition and Human Needs, June 1977) in the following statement:

> The early symptoms of lead poisoning are subtle, subjective and non specific and therefore not so readily recognised in children . . . In children such mild symptoms are often overlooked or attributed to other disease states, so that poisoning due to lead is more likely to be recognised first at a late or severe stage on the basis of nervous system involvement (acute encephalopathy).

A QUICK ANTI-POLLUTION GUIDE

Many of the effects of pollution can be eliminated, avoided or at least counteracted by sensible approaches and proper nutrition. Following are some alternatives to pollutants used in the home and some ways to help reduce the effect pollutants have on your body.

(Cont.)

A Quick Anti-Pollution Guide (Cont.)

- Everybody (especially pregnant women and breastfeeding mothers) should try to avoid using pesticides in the home. Pests can be eliminated, or at least minimised, by the judicious use of herbs. Cat thyme, for example, acts as a broad-spectrum insect repellant. The crushed leaves of pennyroyal will help to keep mosquitoes away and tansy tends to repel flies.

- Vitamin C supplement helps neutralise the effects of nitrates in foods by blocking the formation of potentially dangerous and carcinogenic nitrosamines. The slow release of Vitamin C affords some degree of protection from meal to meal and from snacks taken during the day.

- Ozone and nitrogen dioxide, common pollutants in western cities, increase the degeneration of lipid components of lung cells and the subsequent formation of free radicals (these are toxic particles formed during certain chemical reactions in the body and are thought to be responsible for ageing, cancer and degenerative diseases).

- Vitamin C and zinc both inhibit the absorption of lead and help the body dispose of it. Vitamin C also promotes all cellular responses to hormones.

- A lack of calcium or Vitamin D_3 predisposes individuals (especially children) to bronchial constriction which causes breathing difficulties such as asthma.

- The more natural your diet, the less stress you place on your body and all bodily functions will benefit.

Another example is that of Brethism, which is a syndrome of mercury intoxication characterised by a cluster of symptoms that mimic the behaviour of a tormented neurotic:

> I had a sore mouth, dizzy spells, and was so weak and tired at night that I found it hard to get my supper and do my work. I was so grouchy and nervous I would cry at nothing . . . I often woke suddenly and had a fluttering feeling like I was scared and floating in space. I was trembly and nervous, and my eyes were bloodshot. I forgot things easily.'

This statement is not from a 'neurotic' but from a woman who was constantly exposed to mercury in an electric motor components factory. Such symptoms remind us that human behaviour reflects the condition of the whole human organism, not just the liver, heart, brain or an enzyme system. As the study of neurotoxins makes clear, it is the whole organism that complains of pains, becomes confused, or gets irritable and depressed. Hopefully further medical research will be addressed to the study of synergism (combined action) and the less obvious causes of disease.

10

BEHAVIOURAL TOXICOLOGY— POLLUTANTS IN OUR ENVIRONMENT

The theory of evolution may not be accepted by everybody but it seems evident that the human body has evolved over millions of years and, during that time, has had to adapt itself to the environment. Originally, although life may have been extraordinarily harsh, the environment was nevertheless quite clean: clean air, a natural diet, plenty of physical activity and a total absence of manufactured, synthetic substances characterised our ecosystem. The changes that have occurred over very long time-spans have allowed for a painstakingly slow, but essential, process of adaptation.

Changes in the environment

In the past few decades we have begun to 'modify' our environment at a frightening and ever-accelerating rate. Dr Bernard Rimland, a world authority on behavioural toxicology, made the following comments in an address on pollution:

> I use the word 'modify' although on first writing I used the word 'violating', then considered alternatives such as 'degrading' or 'poisoning' before settling on the ostensibly neutral term 'modify'. I hope my message gets across.

Modern industry is now using more than 100,000 chemicals of which approximately 650 have already been declared dangerous by the United States government in their Toxics Release Inventory (TRI). Several other countries, including the UK, Canada, Australia and Japan, have also produced Pollutant or Toxic Release Inventories, and an initial list of Persistent Organic Pollutants (POPs) to be banned has now been agreed by the United Nations.

While it is true that many of these chemicals need to be present in reasonably large amounts before they affect our health, there are also some that can cause serious problems at very low levels of exposure.

Most, if not all, chemicals can interact with one another so that their effect becomes greater than the sum of their parts. This is called the 'synergistic effect'. In practical terms, it simply means that when combined, these can damage our health even at levels considered totally harmless for any of the chemicals alone.

An individual may be capable of coping with two very late nights each and every week, without affecting his work output. The same individual may also have the flu once or twice each year, again without suffering any substantial ill-effects. But what about if he has the flu and two consecutive late nights? It may just be too much!

Different types of pollution

The science that deals with the effects of toxic chemicals on human behaviour is named behavioural toxicology and it is an integral part of orthomolecular medicine and psychiatry.

Among the thousands of cases we see and treat at the Complementary and Environmental Medicine Centre, a considerable proportion of so-called 'psychiatric' or 'behavioural' problems, especially among children, are found to be directly or indirectly related to some form of 'pollution'. I give this word the same meaning as Dr Rimland:

Polluted air and water are all too well known. The lesser-known forms, usually not even considered to be manifestations of pollution, are to an increasing degree turning out to be important causes of mental and physical handicap in the human population, especially when the impact occurs during the prenatal or early developmental stages.

Nutritional pollution includes sins of both omission and commission. It includes the omission from the diet of crucially important vitamins and minerals, especially Vitamin C, the B vitamins, as well as Vitamin E and such minerals as magnesium, iron and zinc. The effects are tragic. Foods supplying these nutrients, which are needed for proper health and development, have been replaced with junk foods, gross and damaging amounts of sugar and other additives that are designed to be attractive to the eye and taste buds, whatever the cost to the rest of the body.

This last statement reminds me of a cartoon I saw once in a magazine which showed a man standing in front of a supermarket shouting, 'Come and get it . . . beautiful foods . . . fresh from the factory!'

Dr Rimland also tells us that we must include in a list of pollution constituents those factors which could be called 'inadvertent'. These forms of pollution include excess copper from water pipes, lead from auto exhausts, pipes, paints, toothpaste tubes and tinned foods, as well as pesticides and plastics.

Then there is the case of medical pollution. According to Dr Rimland medically prescribed and over-the-counter drugs kill more people than breast cancer while some fifty million hospital-patient days per year are attributable to drug 'side-effects' in the United States. And that was in 1975!

Living organisms have a considerable capacity for adaptation and the human organism has indeed adapted in many ways. For example, as we chew less raw food, our mandibles and teeth have undergone considerable changes, but our capacity to adapt is far from infinite and requires long periods of time.

We all inherit some limitations regarding what foods we can eat. Some of us, for example, lack the suitable enzymes to digest milk, others acquire limitations for various reasons, ranging from self-imposed restrictions due to religious beliefs through to degenerative diseases like diabetes.

Quite apart from these specific limitations, we live in a world which has enough natural poisons without having to cope with the considerable amounts of 'chemical poisons' we have introduced thus making life even more hazardous than it would naturally be.

Environmental poisons and toxicology

Traditionally, toxicology deals with the immediate effects—including death—attributable, directly or indirectly, to ingestion or contact with a poison. However, as a scientific approach, toxicology is not without flaws.

To begin with, most substances are tested singly. The effect of each separate substance is noted but no allowance is made for the fact that the combined effect of two or three or more chemicals may be quite different from that of a single one. And, when you think of it, this is plain common sense. Mix any two foods or drinks and you get a taste that is often quite different from that of any of its constituents.

Food additives are tested to see if they produce pathological changes in animals. Blood defects, developmental rates and certain crucial physiological parameters, such as liver functions, may be examined. From such studies, toxicologists calculate quantities of one single substance that can be ingested without causing any measurable abnormality. The resulting figure is then divided by ten to allow for differences among various species, and again by ten for human safety.

This then becomes the allowable daily intake for humans. However, the effects, if any, on the behaviour of these animals is almost never measured. Dr David Ball, director of the National Institute for Environmental Health Sciences in Australia, is fond of pointing out that if the effect of thalidomide had been to lower the capacity for academic ability by, say, 10 per cent, it would never have been detected.

There is also another very important flaw in the way we test the toxicity of most potential pollutants. Humans are exposed to, and consume, a large amount of chemicals and additives (colourings, preservatives and so on). The exposed population includes the very young, the very old, the healthy and the infirm. It also includes the constitutionally strong as well as people with disabilities or predispositions—genetic or otherwise—that may render them more susceptible than others.

Some may have a degree of exposure which is far greater than average. Schoolchildren are much more likely to eat large amounts of colouring agents from lollies, ice blocks, soft drinks and similar foods, than adults. Because they are shorter, and therefore closer to the ground, they are exposed to greater amounts of lead pollution from car exhausts than adults. Their metabolic rate, and the fact that they tend to be in constant physical motion, also makes lead all the more dangerous for them. At least until a certain age, they are more likely to place dirty and dusty objects, including their fingers, into their mouths.

However, when a substance is being tested by a toxicologist, the usual procedure is to choose a group of healthy animals, quite similar to each other in age, who are then fed a similar and nutritious diet. These are then challenged with one *single* agent.

The results are bound to be quite different when an average cross-section of the population, including the young and old people on different diets, is exposed to dozens, even hundreds of substances *simultaneously*.

THE CASE OF TARTRAZINE

When a group of rats was exposed to tartrazine (yellow) additives, those who were fed a diet which was perfectly balanced in respect to proteins, carbohydrates, vitamins and minerals but 'purified' were very badly affected. The yellow additive was in fact toxic to them.

When the *same* additive was given to a group of rats fed on a natural diet, such as they would normally obtain in their environment, the animals showed no ill effects, although that diet may not have been as perfectly balanced as the purified, supplemented one. Apparently the difference was caused by the fact that the first diet did not supply fibres!

11

ALCOHOL

'Beer makes you feel the way you ought to feel without beer.' So said the great Australian writer, Henry Lawson. This statement applies to any kind of alcohol not just beer, because, after all, alcohol is a mood-altering drug.

In moderation, alcohol makes most people feel happy, it can be lots of fun and it can also aid digestion, help to prevent heart disease and perhaps even help you live a little longer—that is, if you drink it in moderation.

There is little doubt that we are getting more and more health conscious and that people are beginning to realise that what you put in your mouth has an enormous bearing on your health. However, when it comes to applying this realisation to alcohol, we stop short. Alcohol consumption in the UK continues to grow steadily and British teenagers are acknowledged to be the heaviest drinkers in Europe. The rise in binge drinking is perhaps the most alarming aspect.

The metabolism of alcohol

Alcohol has been with us since time immemorial. A special enzyme with the exclusive task of breaking down alcohol exists in the human liver. This enzyme is called alcohol dehydrogenase and it probably evolved to enable primitive man to digest fermented fruit fallen to the ground in prehistoric forests.

ALCOHOL AND THE ECONOMY

In the 1999–2000 financial year the UK government collected £6426 million in customs and excise revenues and £5073.8 million in VAT from the sale of beer, wine and spirits. The total of £11,499.8 million represented 4.4 per cent of the total revenue collected in taxes for that year.

The alcohol industry is estimated to spend about £270 million a year in advertising to promote the sale of beer, wine and spirits.

Alcohol is very big business. It has political clout. It employs thousands of people and it kills thousands every year, indirectly through road crashes and insidiously as the result of chronic disease.

The effects of alcohol are caused by a mood-altering and toxic substance called ethyl alcohol. It is a clear and volatile substance that is formed by the action of yeast on fruit juices and there is about one tablespoon of ethyl alcohol in a standard Britishbeer.

Ethyl alcohol dissolves in both water and fat and reaches practically every organ in the body (including the spinal column, brain cells and bones) within a few minutes of being ingested. The results of drinking depend not so much on the quantity of alcohol drunk but on the amount of ethyl alcohol that reaches the bloodstream and how quickly it gets there. The faster it gets into the bloodstream, the more potent are its effects.

Roughly 5 per cent of what you drink is absorbed directly from the stomach into the bloodstream and the remainder passes through a living 'valve' called the pyloric sphincter before ending up in the small intestine, where it is also absorbed into the bloodstream.

The pylorus is a muscular ring which contracts when the chemical composition of the foodstuffs in the stomach is inappropriate, or when there is too much food. If the pylorus can be kept shut, or only slightly open, this will slow down the movement of alcohol. Therefore, alcohol taken on an empty stomach moves through quickly, and its effects are quite powerful—as every drinker knows only too well.

Food delays the absorption of alcohol considerably irrespective of whether it is eaten before or with the drink. Fatty, oily foods are especially valuable in slowing down the movement of alcohol through the pyloric sphincter.

Sparkling wines, champagne or spirits with soda contain carbon dioxide and the bubbles 'tickle' the pylorus, causing it to open. This is one of the reasons why you can get quite drunk on a relatively weak beverage, such as spumante.

After alcohol reaches the blood it goes to the liver, then to the heart and lungs. It then races through the entire body, eventually getting to the brain where it stimulates the production of endorphins which act as an anaesthetic.

The only way to get sober is to get the alcohol out of the blood; and you can only do this via urine, breath, sweat and by liver action. Although it may seem more, only about 3 per cent of alcohol leaves via the urine and around 5 per cent leaves via sweat and breath. The rest has to be broken down (oxidised) by the liver. It takes about one hour for the liver to dispose of the alcohol contained in one standard drink. The liver has to be in good condition to do this and it should not be already overburdened with taking care of other toxins.

How the liver deals with alcohol

The liver is the only organ that does not get its energy from blood sugar; it uses proteins instead. For the liver to function properly it needs a good balance of proteins, vitamins and minerals.

Often alcoholics have an unbalanced diet that is high in calories but poor in nutrients and proteins, which means that the liver has to work overtime to clear large amounts of alcohol without having the necessary proteins and nutrients for optimal function.

Because alcohol is high in calories, a heavy drinker may satisfy most, if not all, of his or her energy needs without eating a thing. For this and other reasons it has always been thought that the many health problems associated with alcoholism were, in fact, caused by malnutrition.

Chronic alcohol consumption can cause irritation and inflammation of the linings of the stomach, intestine and pancreas which severely impairs the absorption of nutrients. It can also impair the liver's ability to handle acetaldehyde which is the principal product of alcohol and a very toxic substance that can cause damage to the liver.

Acetaldehyde interferes with the activation of vitamins by the liver cells and the enzyme responsible for breaking down alcohol in the liver, alcohol dehydrogenase, seems to be dependent on Vitamin C. This has been described as the metabolic trap suffered by many alcoholics. Many scientists also believe that it is acetaldehyde which is responsible for the effects of alcohol on the heart, the brain and the dependence caused by the drinking in the first place.

ALCOHOL ADDICTION

Alcohol is broken down into acetaldehyde. Acetaldehyde may bind to several of the brain's neurotransmitters and form complexes that act as 'pseudo-transmitters'.

One of the reactions of these pseudo-transmitters is to form endorphins, the brain's own natural opiates, which explains the ability of alcohol to reduce pain and produce pleasant sensations.

Unfortunately, it also points to one of the reasons why alcohol is so addictive: if acetaldehyde increases the production of opiates in the brain, it is easy to see why one would become addicted to its effects. This is much the same as the way joggers become addicted to endorphins and gamblers to adrenalin.

Liver cells get rid of the excess hydrogen formed by alcohol, by shunting it into the formation of alphaglycerophosphates and fatty acids. These are the precursors of triglycerides, notoriously implicated in both liver damage and heart and circulatory disorders.

A condition, known as hyperlipaemia, is now established as one of the major predisposing factors in cardiovascular disease and one that is entirely correctable simply by avoiding alcohol.

Alcohol also competes with other drugs for detoxification so that their metabolism is slowed down and any of their dangerous effects enhanced. This is why alcohol can kill when mixed with some medications, especially tranquillisers.

Is it only alcoholics who suffer liver damage from alcohol?

Charles Lieber carried out an interesting experiment which he reported in *Scientific American* (1976, Vol. 234, No. 3, p. 25). A group of volunteers were fed a good, low-fat diet in which proteins accounted for 25 per cent of calories. They were also given ample vitamin and mineral supplements. They were asked to drink six standard drinks per day for eighteen days.

Routine thin-needle biopsy revealed a progressive rise in liver fat after only a few days and by the end of the eighteen days the increase was in the order of eightfold! There were also striking changes in the mitochondria (enlargement and distortion) while the sites of enzymes associated with the metabolism of alcohol (smooth membranes of the endoplasmic reticulum) proliferated.

It is for this, and other reasons, that some heavy drinkers show a temporary increase in their capacity to metabolise alcohol so that for a while, perhaps many years, they can drink everybody else 'under the table'.

These changes occurred following a moderate intake of alcohol by a group of healthy, well fed people who at no stage showed any symptoms of intoxication. Drunkenness is not necessary to suffer liver damage!

The effects of alcohol

The effects of alcohol are both physiological and psychological. Following are some of the major physiological effects.

Physiological effects

- Alcohol enlarges blood vessels so that you tend to feel warmer. This is only an illusion, however, because alcohol actually enhances heat losses and therefore lowers your resistance to cold weather. Dilated blood vessels can often be seen on the nose and cheeks of heavy drinkers.
- Alcohol affects blood pressure. If you suffer from high blood pressure and drink more than five drinks per day (two

ALCOHOL 177

drinks per day for women), you are wasting your time getting treatment for high blood pressure as the alcohol pushes the blood pressure up anyway.

- Cardiomyopathy, an irreversible weakening of the heart muscle, can be caused by excess alcohol. However, it has been shown that moderate drinking can dilate coronary arteries and therefore relieve high blood pressure, thus lowering the risk of coronary thrombosis. This paradoxical effect may explain why statistics show that moderate drinkers die of heart attacks less often than those who don't drink at all.

- Alcohol can cause gastritis—chronic inflammation and thickening of the stomach lining. It can also affect the lining of the intestine and the pancreas.

- Alcohol causes various problems in the liver. See the section on 'How the liver deals with alcohol'.

- Alcohol has been associated with an increased risk of cancer in the upper respiratory and digestive systems. Heavy drinkers often smoke a lot which compounds the risk of getting cancer.

- Alcohol leads to biochemical abnormalities which have many effects on physiology. Among them are:

  1. An increase in lactate which can cause periods of severe anxiety in susceptible individuals.
  2. A decrease in ketosteroids, which can affect sex hormones and create imbalances between various hormones.
  3. A decreased tolerance to galactose (a milk sugar).
  4. A decrease in oxidation of amines which can lead to abnormal ratios of important brain chemicals.
  5. An increase in fat deposits.
  6. Inhibition of blood-sugar formation via gluconeogenesis thus diminishing energy reserves for the body and the brain.
  7. Changes to the energy production of cells.
  8. Elevation of uric acid levels.
  9. Decreased protein synthesis that can slow down the repair mechanisms of the body.
  10. Protein and fat retention in the liver.
  11. Depression of glutathione, an antioxidant component necessary in the removal of free radicals.

12. The stimulation of alcohol metabolism by the liver (smooth endoplasmic reticulum) so that, for a while, a person seems to be able to hold his alcohol.

Psychological effects

Alcohol dulls pain and depresses those centres in the brain that are responsible for controlling behaviour. It lowers inhibitions so that we no longer feel anxious, guilty or foolish when we behave in an outlandish fashion. Another common effect of alcohol is to make people depressed. The psychological effects of alcohol are very diverse and depend, to a great extent, on the individual.

ALCOHOLISM AND HEREDITY

We now have good evidence that there is a strong inheritance factor in alcoholism and that an addictive substance is actually produced by the brain of people who drink regularly.

Studies show that when the children of alcoholics are adopted by other families, they are just as likely to become alcoholics as are those reared by their biological parents. In other words it would seem that nature could turn out to be stronger than nurture.

Alcohol and nutrition

Is it true that alcohol is good for the digestion? Yes and no! Alcohol tends to inhibit some of the enzymes for the breakdown of food but, if taken in moderation or diluted, it can stimulate the secretion of gastric juices which help the digestion of proteins. To achieve that effect, however, you don't necessarily have to drink alcohol, just the smell of it or even some fumes will get the digestive juices flowing.

Biochemical changes, which vary from individual to individual, dictate exactly what kind of effect alcohol will have on you. If you are the type that becomes a little anxious after drinking, the easiest way to avoid this happening is to take some calcium on an empty stomach well before you start drinking, and then some more while you are drinking.

If you are prone to becoming a little depressed when drinking, take some Vitamin C with a little zinc, in powder form. These will help to speed up the breakdown of alcohol. Another way to help your body get rid of alcohol a little more quickly is to drink large amounts of fruit sugar (fructose). The best way, of course, is with fruit juices.

Of course you can take something that will slow down your desire to drink. Vitamin B_3 in the niacin or nicotinic acid form is reported to do this. Please note that Vitamin B_3 may cause a severe flushing effect. Although this in itself is not harmful, it may frighten you. Some allergic people can have a severe skin rash following the intake of niacin and, if so, should avoid it. Another nutrient that is said to decrease the craving for alcohol and that helps you to remain sober is the common amino acid, glutamic acid.

The controversial supplement, Vitamin B_{15} (pangamic acid), is said to decrease or even reverse some of the effects of alcohol on the liver. The Russians have been using it for years and swear by it.

ALLERGIES AND ALCOHOL

If you are allergic to some foods and are on a special diet, remember that alcoholic beverages fall into three categories: spirits, wines and beers.

Spirits are a fermentation of wheat, barley or potatoes; wines are made from grapes which need no added yeast because their skin has a natural yeast; and beers are made of barley and yeast, with or without hops.

The hangover

If you are only a moderate drinker, a session with a half a dozen drinks may give you a nasty time the morning after. The symptoms of a hangover vary greatly among individuals but can include any of the following: vomiting, loss of appetite, headache, sleeplessness, tiredness, a loss of balance and/or co-ordination, thirst, and a feeling that your muscles and joints are not up to the job of supporting and propelling you anywhere further than the nearest armchair. The reasons for all this are:

- You have drunk more than your liver has been able to cope with and get rid of and the extra alcohol is still circulating around in your blood.
- Alcohol blocks the stress signals so that as the brain 'wakes up' in the morning it starts to receive all the stress signals at once. It finds it hard to cope with so much so suddenly.

Although some people get headaches from drinking any alcohol, certain wines, especially the red ones, seem to affect people more often than others. They contain histamine and this chemical can cause headaches in susceptible people. Some researchers think the tannins (which give wines body and astringent properties) are more likely to be the culprits. Sulphur dioxide, used as an additive and preservative, may also be responsible because it can cause bronchial constriction. It is certainly unhealthy for asthmatics!

More recently, it has been discovered that substances called congeners, which provide most of the taste, smell and colour of different drinks, may be an important factor in alcohol-related headaches. Congeners are made up from wood alcohol and fuel oil, both of which are very toxic even in relatively small amounts. They can cause blindness and enlarge the arteries of the brain in much the same way as histamines are said to do. Vodka is a drink that is low in congeners while whisky, brandy and red wines have a high content of congeners.

Mixing drinks (there is always some scientific truth in old wives' tales!) is tantamount to mixing and increasing total congeners. Hence, the hangovers tend to become fiercer as the cocktails become more exotic. So, if you are having a great night out and sample a little of that delicate white wine, and some of the gutsy red, plus a little pre-dinner cocktail, with a brandy after dinner, the chances are your hangover will be worse than if you kept to one type of drink. One of the solutions to reducing hangovers is to drink the same beverage and to choose ones that are low in congeners—these usually have less aroma.

Thirst   Thirst is a common result of drinking. It is not, however, caused by dehydration but by an unhealthy rearrangement of your body fluids. Alcohol causes water to spill out of cells and into the extracellular fluid thus making you thirsty and causing some extra pressure in your head. This phenomenon will also make your eyes look red and bloodshot in the morning.

Sleep   Alcohol interferes with rapid eye movement (REM) sleep which is essential for the recuperating period to have a positive effect. Without a reasonable amount of REM sleep one tends to be tired, irritable and anxious.

One of the simplest insurances for drinkers is to take a multimineral-multivitamin tablet plus some Vitamin B_1 (thiamine) every day. According to one leading neurologist who is a world authority on the effects of alcohol on the brain, Professor Byron Kakulas, head of the Department of Neuropathology at Royal Perth Hospital in Australia, 'many of the effects of alcohol can be nullified by taking a few vitamins, especially thiamine which would immediately reduce one of the most common organic mental disorders associated with alcohol'.

How to decrease the effects of hangovers

- Alcohol is a diuretic, so drink lots of fluids before and after imbibing.
- Drink some fruit juices as this will help your overworked liver metabolise acetaldehyde a little faster.
- Take some B-complex vitamins, perhaps with a dash of antacid.
- Eat before and while you are drinking as this slows down the absorption of the alcohol. Milk, fats and oils line the stomach while starches absorb some of the alcohol.
- Have some Vitamin C as this not only helps to absorb the alcohol but it also helps the liver to break down the alcohol.
- Avoid drinking several different types of alcohol or alcohols that have high amounts of congeners.
- Stay up for an extra couple of hours after you finish drinking and sleep late.
- According to research in America, the oil of evening primrose is said to prevent and cure hangovers.

How to break the alcohol cycle

Drug therapy

Propranolol, a beta blocker used in the treatment of high blood pressure and anxiety, has been suggested as suitable medication for alcoholics. When taken together with alcohol, propranolol seems to block the mood-altering effects of liquor.

As most people drink expecting a change in the way they feel, they may reduce, or stop, their alcohol intake when no such change occurs. It is also possible that the anxiety-reducing effects of the drug may play a role as many people suspect it is one of the factors which drives people to drink in the first place.

Be that as it may, there seems to be a considerable amount of evidence suggesting that the outcome of treatment of alcoholism is not significantly affected by the form of treatment used. A comprehensive American study, called the Rand report (*New Scientist*, December 1983, p. 749) concluded that:

> Perhaps the most important finding . . . is that there are few noteworthy differences among remission rates for various treatment types. Regardless of the setting in which treatment occurs, remissions appear quite uniform, fluctuating by 100 per cent at most . . . despite the manifest differences in philosophy, organisation and treatment procedures among the sample centres.

However, some forms of treatment not covered by the Rand report demand a degree of attention.

Nutritional supplements

Niacin

Russell Smith is an American physician who has been involved in the treatment of alcoholics in American hospitals since the 1940s. In 1973, and again in 1978, he completed and reported (*Journal of Orthomolecular Psychiatry*, 1978, Vol. 7, No. 1, p. 53) on the results of a five-year study with five hundred diagnosed alcoholics who were treated with large doses of Vitamin B_3 in the form of nicotinic acid (niacin):

Nicotinamide (another form of Vitamin B_3) proved of no value to alcoholics, suggesting perhaps another mechanism of action. Nicotinic acid improved sleep patterns, mood stability and overall functioning in 60 per cent of the test group who showed the more serious organic symptoms of the disease. Nicotinic acid significantly reduced acquired tolerance to alcohol and appeared to shorten the course of the acute toxic brain syndrome while all but eliminating the 'dry drunk syndrome': hyperexcitable manic episodes and serious, potentially suicidal depression.

Nicotinic acid crosses the blood-brain barrier easily and tends to inhibit tryptamine while reducing the levels of serotonin and dopamine. Elevated brain levels of these two chemicals have been associated with psychiatric disorders and behavioural abnormalities.

Noradrenaline levels may also be suppressed by nicotinic acid but, more importantly, Smith suggests that nicotinic acid can stimulate histamine and act as a governor of brain catecholamines in general. Histamine itself tends to inhibit monoamine oxidase reactions, a factor which could account for its mood-elevating properties and anti-depressant activity. I have used niacin therapy as part of my treatment of alcoholics with considerable success.

THE HAIR OF THE DOG

Does the hair of the dog help with hangovers? Having a drink the next morning will help a hangover because the methanol enzymes prefer ethanol. So one more drink will shift their attention, so to speak, away from methanol and less of its nasty by-products will be formed—for a while at least.

Histamine, vitamins, minerals and dietary manipulations

Dr Oscar Kruesi, of the Huxley Institute for Bio Social Research, New York, has developed another approach to alcoholism which is based on regulating histamine levels with vitamins, minerals and dietary manipulations.

We have known for some time that histamine may be a neuro-transmitter: two of the world's leading experts on brain biochemistry, Snyder and Axelford, claim it is but we had to wait for Dr Carl Pfeiffer, of the New Jersey Neuropsychiatric Institute, for confirmation of this fact during the 1970s.

There are, in the human body, two separate histamine receptors: H_1 and H_2. H_1 involves well established allergic responses and H_2 is a brain histamine receptor (*Nature*, 1982, Vol. 272, p. 329).

Pfeiffer discovered that there are two groups of alcoholics which have either very high or very low histamine levels. In the treatment of alcoholism it is very important to know to which group the patient belongs. For information about the high and low histamine levels, see page 38.

Alcohol and its effect on the brain

Dr Jean Lennane, past director of Drug and Alcohol Services at Rozelle and Gladesville Psychiatric Hospital in Australia, conducted research into the extent of alcohol-related brain damage in people who regularly consume alcohol.

In 1983 the *Sun Herald* reported that 'Australians drink an average of 2.4 drinks per man, woman and child every day of their lives'. Dr Lennane estimates that considering children don't usually drink and that 15 per cent of adults are teetotallers, the rest must drink a lot more than 2.4 glasses.

Two hundred cases had been assessed up to April 1983 and the youngest case reported was a 34-year-old journalist who after having four drinks per day for ten years and one final binge, ended up in hospital with severe frontal lobe damage and impaired memory. The condition of this patient is irreversible.

Dr Lennane is careful with her pronouncements: 'Not every social drinker will suffer brain damage. Some people are more tolerant than others. The danger is we don't know yet who is at risk.' Often, it is not the alcoholic or the derelict on skid row that we should worry about but the ordinary person who steadily consumes alcohol every day.

ALCOHOL AND OSTEOPOROSIS

Women who drink large amounts of alcohol are ten times more likely to develop osteoporosis. Calcium supplements will not help if you drink more than one bottle of beer per day, or its equivalent, according to Dr Richard Evans of the Metabolic Unit of the Concord Hospital in Sydney.

Dr Lennane suggests that anyone who has eight or more drinks per day should have an assessment of his or her ability to function normally.

Loss of adaptability

The frontal lobes of the brain are often affected by alcohol. At worst, people affected by alcohol have a great deal of difficulty in organising simple tasks, or lack the incentive to do anything. At best, their organising skills which depend on frontal lobes are diminished.

Frontal lobe damage is insidious because people still retain their normal intelligence but lose the ability to work out whether they have a problem or not—let alone do something about it. Many people don't realise this until they are presented with a new set of problems which demand the ability to adjust.

ALCOHOL THE DRUG

Alcohol is a drug in every sense of the word. It is, in fact, a mood-altering drug with profound short- and long-term effects on almost every part of the human body and most facets of human physiology, particularly on the biochemistry of the brain. If alcohol were discovered today and a pharmaceutical company tried to market it, I doubt that it would be allowed without a doctor's prescription!

The habitual drinker loses his capacity to adapt. As little as a couple of drinks per day over some years can cause chronic impairment of intelligence. Drinking can cause the brain to actually shrink because of cell death. This results in memory loss, decreased intelligence, impairment of thinking and alterations to personality.

Impaired intelligence

One feature of intelligence that may suffer as a result of chronic alcohol consumption, perhaps even at moderate or 'social drinking' levels, is crystallised intelligence. This is defined as the ability to use an accumulated body of general information to make judgements and solve problems.

In practical terms, crystallised intelligence is that used in understanding the various facets of an argument, the real meaning of newspaper editorials or in dealing with problems for which there are no clear answers but only better or worse options. By the time one arrives at that stage, however, it is often too late for total recovery.

SOME OF THE BENEFITS OF ALCOHOL

Statistical studies have shown that moderate drinkers tend to live slightly longer than teetotallers, longer than ex-drinkers and longer than people who drink more than three to four drinks per day.

- Drinking with meals seems to help the digestion. Perhaps the alcohol stimulates the protein-splitting enzymes. It may also put the drinker in a good mood, something which in itself favours good food assimilation, higher immune resistance and better blood circulation.
- Blood pressure was found to be lowest among people who drink three or fewer drinks per day. However, it increases progressively with each drink after that and almost doubles at six or more drinks per day.
- The key to minimising the bad effects of drinking appears to be to drink with meals, and then, to drink only in moderation—no more than two to three glasses of wine per day.

12

THE CHEMISTRY OF LOVE

There is sex and there is love, and there is love without sex and sex without love as well as sexual love. Everybody knows what being colour blind means and it may surprise you that there is a disease which causes some people to become 'love blind'.

Such people are normal in every respect: they may be very friendly, sociable individuals who often form close relationships with members of the opposite sex and may even get married, but they cannot experience the intense feeling of passion known as 'being in love' any more than a colour-blind person can discern the brilliant shades and hues of a colourful painting.

As humanity moves away from its poetic and religious past towards the robotic future of the 21st century, we are discovering that love blindness is only one of the many psycho-sexual problems that stem, at least in part, from neuroendocrinological fluctuations and imbalances. Loss of libido, separation anxiety, hysteroid dysphoria, delusional love, dependence syndrome, paranoid jealousy, hypo-manic love and obsessive infatuation are some of the new labels believed to be closely linked with the deranged brain biochemistry of some interpersonal relationships.

Being in love is one of the most intense personal experiences possible and, like most of our moods, there are some chemical changes within our brains that are associated with it. Anyone who has ever been in love knows that it is a state somewhat reminiscent of madness, hyperactivity and hallucination.

According to Dr Michael Liebowitz, a neurophysiologist of Columbia University, New York, there are three basic types of love:

1. There is the adrenalin kind which is characterised by the orgasmic, hedonistic pursuit of sexual arousal and fulfilment.
2. There is romantic love in which the brain manufactures large quantities of a group of chemicals called 'enkephalines' which can lessen the sensation of pain but may also be responsible for hallucinations, delusions and a remarkable inability to think clearly.
3. There is 'marital love', which is thought to be associated with an increased production of natural opiates (a group of morphine-like substances which dull the senses) in the brain.

The brain's natural opiates

When you are in love, you feel 'high' and you may have noticed the similarity between the withdrawal symptoms associated with the break-up of relationships and those elicited by amphetamine withdrawal.

One of the reasons for this is that an 'in love' brain manufactures more phenylethylalanine, a chemical derived from a common, everyday amino acid found in many foods, phenylalanine. As soon as an affair starts to turn sour the brain halts, or drastically reduces, its output of phenylethylalanine and the person involved begins to suffer withdrawal symptoms.

Dr Donald Klein and Dr Michael Liebowitz conducted an in-depth study of such people and found that a considerable number of them tended to go on a chocolate binge as soon as they began to suffer some of the depression associated with the break-up of their relationship. Why chocolate? Because this gastronomic delight is extracted from the seeds of *Theobroma cacao* (which literally means 'food of the gods') and its main constituent, theobromine, is a stimulant. It is also rich in phenylalanine.

Phenylalanine is also used by the brain to make norepinephrine (noradrenaline) and to slow down the breakdown of natural opiates (the endorphins and enkephalines) which are responsible for, among other things, lowering the sensation of pain. An increased intake of phenylalanine may result in higher brain levels of endorphins and therefore a decreased sensitivity to pain. So it stands to reason that phenylalanine could be useful as a sort of 'natural' painkiller or antidepressant.

The pain of being in love, if the love is not reciprocated or the affair is terminated, can be as debilitating as any psychiatric illness and it may well be that phenylalanine, or chocolate, could be used by lovers to reduce the intensity of their love-sickness.

Foods containing phenylalanine

almonds	egg
apple	fish (herring)
avocado	milk
baked beans	parsley
banana	peanuts
beef	pineapple
beet	soya bean
carrot	soy proteins
chicken	spinach
cottage cheese	tomato
chocolate	

Hormone stimulation

The hypothalamus is in charge of our behaviour in general and our sexual tendencies in particular. This small portion of the brain which is also known as a 'neuroendocrinal transducer' translates inputs (transducing) from our external and internal environments into special chemicals known as 'releasing factors' that are a type of hormone. These in turn travel to the pituitary gland and cause it to release its various hormones, which are then circulated to reach the various endocrine glands which, thus stimulated, begin to pour out their hormones.

In simple terms, when a man looks into the eyes of the woman he loves, what he sees is first changed from light impulses to electrical pulsations. These move along the optic nerves and reach the brain where they are again transformed by the hypothalamus into releasing factors which eventually cause adrenal hormones to make his heart beat faster. This can also happen with olfactory stimulation by the subtle, often barely discernible, pheromones. Though the influence of scents on sexual behaviour is not recognised at a conscious level, other stimulants can produce dramatic effects and it may well be that people with blockages along one of these circuits turn out to be love-blind.

People suffering with decreased pituitary function (hypopituitarism) often have problems with their feelings. However, in sexual matters, it is the hypothalamus which sends luteinising hormone releasing factors (LHRF) to the pituitary which then pours out two separate hormones, follicle stimulating hormone (FSH) and luteinising hormone (LH). FSH instructs the testes to start sperm production and LH is responsible for the production of testosterone—the male sex hormone.

While it might seem that the hypothalamus is responsible for fuelling sexual encounters, perhaps it is the brain's own opiates (phenylalanine) that may be responsible for keeping couples together.

People may cling desperately to their partner to keep up their production of phenylethylalanine and therefore avoid withdrawal. Perhaps they are unwittingly using their partner as a mood regulator!

However, like anything, too much of a good thing can be harmful, and excessive amounts of the brain's own opiates can cause people to become insensitive or dulled to physical and emotional interaction.

CHOCOLATE ADDICTION

So pleasant is the stimulation from chocolate that some people use it almost as a drug. During the 16th century the Spanish government, under pressure from the Church which disapproved of anyone being 'stimulated', banned chocolate because it claimed that it was 'a drink of the devil!'

(Cont.)

Chocolate Addiction (Cont.)

Like prohibitions on all mood-altering substances ever discovered, the only effect this had was to spread its use further and make it more desirable and expensive.

In the ancient markets of Mexico chocolate was actually used as currency. The courtesans of Louis XV used it as a sexual stimulant and more recently *Cosmopolitan* magazine voted it among the top ten aphrodisiacs.

In a sense, however, chocolate may be considered a drug and, like all drugs, it can cause addiction if taken too often. This, of course, gives rise to the depression of withdrawal when it is not available.

Aphrodisiacs

Mankind's search for aphrodisiacs has driven people to swathe themselves in colourful clothes and exotic scents. They have eaten anything that even remotely resembles a sex organ (bananas, oysters and rhinoceros horn) as well as the actual sex organs of animals.

Luteinising hormone releasing factor (LHRF) has been dubbed 'the ultimate aphrodisiac'. This followed reports that its effects are highly specific to sexual behaviour. Robert Moss, Professor of Physiology at the University of Texas Health Science Center in Dallas, has reported that it seems to improve the sexual functioning of some impotent males.

LHRF has also been tested as a contraceptive for both males and females and it has been found that while it enhances female libido, there may be some cases where the opposite is true for males.

Dopamine, a neurotransmitter partially involved in sex, is made from tyrosine, a common amino acid now available as a food supplement. However, too much dopamine can be responsible for certain mental illnesses.

Serotonin, made from tryptophan, excites her but can depress his sex drive. Eggs, lecithin and choline, helped along by Vitamin B_1, can help the synthesis of acetylcholine and researchers at Tulane University, New Orleans, claim acetylcholine can have dramatic effects on human sexual behaviour.

Meanwhile, would-be Romeos may try the local fruit shop. While various perfume makers have been desperately trying to find a sex-attractant scent, the spray-on aphrodisiac, researchers have been looking at androsterone, a potent male hormone which is said to attract females faster than a gleaming red Porsche.

The lowly vegetable, celery, apparently contains some androsterone and it is released through perspiration after digestion. People, I am told, find it irresistible, although it is not detected consciously and I am not sure whether your partner will want to cuddle or nibble you after a celery binge, but it may well be a healthier and sexier alternative to expensive perfume!